Basic
Mathematics
—for the—
Health-Related
Professions

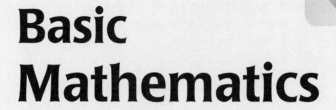

Basic
Mathematics
—for the—
Health-Related
Professions

Lorraine J. Doucette, MS, MT(ASCP), CLS(NCA)
Faculty
School of Health Professions, Wellness and Physical Education
Anne Arundel Community College
Arnold, Maryland

W.B. SAUNDERS COMPANY
A Harcourt Health Sciences Company
Philadelphia London New York St. Louis Toronto Sydney

W.B. SAUNDERS COMPANY
A Harcourt Health Sciences Company

The Curtis Center
Independence Square West
Philadelphia, Pennsylvania 19106

Library of Congress Cataloging-in-Publication Data

Doucette, Lorraine J.
    Basic mathematics for the health-related professions /
Lorraine J. Doucette.
        p. cm.
    ISBN 0–7216–7938–2
    1. Medicine—Mathematics I. Title.
R853.M3 D68 2000
510′.2461—dc21

99–049765

Associate Acquisitions Editor: Shirley A. Kuhn
Associate Developmental Editor: Rachael Zipperlen
Editorial Assistant: Katherine Macciocca
Senior Illustrator: Matt Andrews

BASIC MATHEMATICS FOR
THE HEALTH-RELATED PROFESSIONS   ISBN 0–7216–7938–2

Printed in the United States of America.

Last digit is the print number: 9   8   7   6   5   4   3   2   1

This book is dedicated to all those health care professionals who struggle with math. May this book help you painlessly solve health-related math problems.

Reviewers

Sharlene Aasen, CMA-C
Globe College/Minnesota School of
    Health Sciences
Oakdale, Minnesota

Brian A. Adrian, PhD
Grand Valley State University
Allendale, Michigan

H. Jan Blake, CMA
Ohio Institute of Photography and
    Technology
Dayton, Ohio

Andrea R. Earby, CMA, RMA, MA
Instructor
Western Career College
San Leandro, California

Jeannette Goodwin, RN, BSN, CMA
Southeast Community College
Lincoln, Nebraska

Audrey Elaine Hentzen, PhD,
    MT(ASCP)
Illinois State University
Normal, Illinois

Martha J. Lake, EdD, MT(ASCP)
University of Arkansas for Medical
    Sciences
Little Rock, Arkansas

Jeanne Lee Avery, BA, CMA, EMT-P
Emily Griffith Opportunity School
Denver, Colorado

Rhonda Myers, RMA(AMT)
Metro Business College
Jefferson City, Missouri

Lisa S. Nagle, CMA, BS Ed
Augusta Technical Institute
Augusta, Georgia

Terry Raynor, BS, CMA, NRHAA
Bryant and Stratton
Hampton, Virginia

Robin Snider-Flohr, MBA, RN, CMA
Jefferson Community College
Steubenville, Ohio

Preface

Basic Mathematics for the Health-Related Professions is designed to be used by students of the health professions, as well as by health care practitioners, to assist in the routine mathematical calculations that they may encounter while caring for patients or analyzing patient samples in a small office laboratory. Because the actual duties of health professionals vary widely in scope, some chapters may be more relevant than others to certain health professionals. Feel free to use the chapters of the book that are applicable to your health field and to your mathematical needs.

At the beginning of the book are six practice tests that are designed to be used by students or health care professionals to determine their base knowledge of health-related mathematical calculations. Educators may want to use these practical tests as a quick assessment tool of their students' mathematical knowledge.

The book is divided into three major sections. In Section 1, Chapters 1 through 6 are mathematics review chapters. The first four chapters cover the most basic of mathematical principles, such as basic arithmetic, significant figures, fractions, ratio and proportion, and systems of measurements. Readers who are proficient in basic mathematics may want to review these chapters quickly and then proceed to the following chapters. Chapters 5 and 6 cover information on dilutions, titers, and solutions, and introduce the student to ratio and proportion calculations. Section 2, Chapters 7 and 8, covers information associated with the interpretation and implementation of medication orders, as well as the necessary mathematical calculations that are involved. The third major section, Chapters 9 through 15, relates to laboratory calculations. The first four chapters in this section cover a particular area of the clinical laboratory, including clinical chemistry, hematology, urinalysis, immunology, and microbiology. Chapters 13 through 15 focus on statistical calculations used in the clinical laboratory, such as standard deviation, as well as calculations associated with quality assurance, quality control, and method comparison.

Because the book is designed to be read by a wide audience, each chapter is divided into three subsections: an overview, examples, and practice problems. Within the overview, the content specific for each chapter is discussed in detail. The many examples in this subsection enable students to master the material and health care professionals to better understand the mathematical concepts.

The second subsection, consisting solely of examples, is designed for both students and health care practitioners. Because the phrase "use it or lose it" can apply to understanding and carrying out mathematical calculations, health care practitioners can use the examples as "templates" for calculations that they have to perform. For example, you have to perform a dilution. It may have been a long time since you last performed one. You vaguely remember how to do it but aren't quite sure. By studying the example section, you can find many examples of dilutions. By using these as "templates," you correctly perform your dilution.

Practice problems comprise the third subsection. Solving these problems reinforces the concepts within each chapter. The answers for the practice problems can be found at the back of the book. For problems that cover more difficult subject matter, some answers will be more detailed than others.

A second color used in the book highlights the answer for each problem and aids in following the steps used to calculate the unknown. When appropriate, the unknown value to be determined is shown as a green X. As the calculation proceeds step-by-step, the color green directs the progress of the calculation.

Enjoy!

Lorraine J. Doucette

Acknowledgments

I would like to acknowledge the support given to me by my husband, Richard, and my two sons, Steven and Kenny. Without their support, this book could not have been written. I would also like to thank Barbara Asplen for her role as technical advisor and friend. In addition, I am grateful to Melissa Vaughn, Lori Foust, Linda Epstein, and Christine Jacobs for their technical expertise, which ensured the accuracy and relevance of this book for health care professionals.

Contents

CHAPTER 5

Dilutions and Titers   97

CHAPTER 6

Calculations Associated with Solutions   115

SECTION
2   Calculations Associated with Drug Dosages

CHAPTER 7

Interpreting Medical Orders   127

CHAPTER 11

Hematology and Immunohematology Laboratories   193

CHAPTER 12

Microbiology Laboratory   215

CHAPTER 13

Quality Assurance in the Clinical Laboratory: Basic Statistical Concepts   223

CHAPTER 14

Quality Assurance and Quality Control in the Clinical Laboratory

247

CHAPTER 15

Instrument and Method Assessment

277

Fundamentals of Mathematical Calculations

Practice Tests

There are six practice tests in this section. The purpose of the tests is to assess a student's or practitioner's competence to perform calculations to solve mathematical problems commonly encountered in the health care field. Educators may want to use these tests as pre- and posttest assessment tools.

The tests and the main purpose of each set of tests are as follows:

- Two tests assess competence in basic mathematical principles.
- Two tests assess competence in medication dosage calculations.
- Two tests assess competence in basic laboratory and statistical calculations.

Answers to the Practice Tests can be found in a separate section at the back of the book.

Upon completion of the practice tests, readers should be able to assess their ability to:

1. Perform basic arithmetic calculations, including addition, subtraction, multiplication, and division with positive and negative numbers.
2. Perform calculations including addition, subtraction, multiplication, and division incorporating rules for rounding numbers to achieve the correct result.
3. Perform calculations (incorporating significant figures and/or scientific notation) including addition, subtraction, multiplication, and division to achieve the correct result.
4. Perform addition, subtraction, multiplication, and division calculations involving simple and/or mixed fractions.
5. Convert among fractions, decimal form, and percentage form.
6. Convert between metric units.
7. Convert between metric and nonmetric units.
8. Calculate the dilution made, given the sample volume and diluent volume, as well as determine the sample and diluent volumes when given the desired dilution to be made.
9. Perform ratio and proportion calculations to determine the concentration of solutes and solvents.

10. Calculate dosage requirements of oral medications in both solid and liquid forms.
11. Calculate parenteral dosage requirements.
12. Perform basic chemistry, hematology, immunology, microbiology, and urinalysis calculations.
13. Calculate basic statistics such as the mean, median, and mode.
14. Calculate standard deviation ranges.

Basic Mathematical Principles

PRACTICE TEST 1

Name: _____

Perform the following calculations:

1. $(-15) + 65$	= X	X	=	_____
2. $(-31) + (-25)$	= X	X	=	_____
3. $42 + 65$	= X	X	=	_____
4. $14 - 10$	= X	X	=	_____
5. $7 - (-12)$	= X	X	=	_____
6. 8×5	= X	X	=	_____
7. $9 \times (-2)$	= X	X	=	_____
8. $45 \div 5$	= X	X	=	_____
9. $120 \div 15$	= X	X	=	_____
10. 35.7×2	= X	X	=	_____
11. $43.52 \div 5.0$	= X	X	=	_____
12. $\frac{1}{2} + \frac{3}{4}$	= X	X	=	_____
13. $1\frac{2}{3} + 2\frac{5}{8}$	= X	X	=	_____
14. $1\frac{1}{5} \times \frac{3}{4}$	= X	X	=	_____
15. $\frac{1}{8} \times \frac{1}{2}$	= X	X	=	_____
16. $\frac{5}{6} \div \frac{1}{4}$	= X	X	=	_____
17. $1\frac{7}{8} \div \frac{1}{3}$	= X	X	=	_____

Convert:

18. $\frac{3}{4}$ to percent form   _____

19. $\frac{3}{4}$ to decimal form   _____

20. 0.52 g = X mg   _____

21. 2.5 mg = X g   _____

22. 250 mL = X L   _____

23. 5 cc = X mL   _____

Convert:

24. 1 pound = X kg   _____

25. 65 inches = X cm   _____

26. If 2 mL of sample is added to 8 mL of diluent, what is the dilution? _____

27. If a 1 to 10 ($^1/_{10}$) dilution was performed, what is the dilution factor? _____

28. A 1 to 5 ($^1/_5$) dilution of serum is required. If 100 μL of serum is available, what are the sample and diluent volumes? _____ SV   _____ DV

29. 500 mL of a 50% EtOH solution is required. On hand is a bottle of 75% EtOH. How much of the 75% EtOH is used to make the new solution? _____

30. 1000 mL of a 10% bleach solution is required. A 20% bleach solution is available. How much of the 20% bleach is used to make the new solution? _____

Basic Mathematical Principles

PRACTICE TEST 2

Name: _____

Perform the following calculations:

1. $(-24) + 43$	= X	X = _____
2. $(-12) + (-4)$	= X	X = _____
3. $12 + 56$	= X	X = _____
4. $24 - 13$	= X	X = _____
5. $5 - (-18)$	= X	X = _____
6. 6×5	= X	X = _____
7. $8 \times (-4)$	= X	X = _____
8. $54 \div 5.0$	= X	X = _____
9. $200 \div 50$	= X	X = _____
10. 77.9×4	= X	X = _____
11. $26.95 \div 3$	= X	X = _____
12. $\frac{1}{4} + \frac{6}{8}$	= X	X = _____
13. $1\frac{7}{8} + 2\frac{1}{6}$	= X	X = _____
14. $1\frac{2}{5} \times \frac{5}{6}$	= X	X = _____
15. $\frac{1}{4} \times \frac{1}{2}$	= X	X = _____
16. $\frac{7}{8} \div \frac{1}{4}$	= X	X = _____
17. $1\frac{7}{8} \div \frac{1}{2}$	= X	X = _____

Convert:

18. $\frac{5}{6}$ to percent form　　　_____

19. 75% to decimal form　　　_____

20. $0.39 \text{ g} = X \text{ mg}$　　　_____

21. $125 \text{ mg} = X \text{ g}$　　　_____

22. $150 \text{ mL} = X \text{ L}$　　　_____

23. $10 \text{ cc} = X \text{ mL}$　　　_____

Convert:

24. 165 pounds = X kg   _____

25. 72 inches = X cm   _____

26. If 1 mL of sample is added to 4 mL of diluent, what is the dilution? _____

27. If a 1 to 5 ($^1/_5$) dilution was performed, what is the dilution factor? _____

28. A 1 to 10 ($^1/_{10}$) dilution of serum is required. If 100 µL of serum is available, what are the sample and diluent volumes? _____ SV   _____ DV

29. 500 mL of a 25% EtOH solution is required. On hand is a bottle of 50% EtOH. How much of the 50% EtOH is used to make the new solution? _____

30. 1000 mL of a 10% bleach solution is required. A 50% bleach solution is available. How much of the 50% bleach is used to make the new solution? _____

Dosage Calculations

PRACTICE TEST 3

Name: _____

Define the following terms:

1. prn = _____

2. qd = _____

3. ac = _____

4. SC = _____

5. qam = _____

6. Ordered: Inderal 10 mg po.
   On hand: Inderal 20 mg per scored tablet.
   How many tablets would you give? _____

7. Ordered: Amoxicillin 500 mg po.
   On hand: Amoxicillin 250 mg per tablet.
   How many tablets would you give? _____

8. Ordered: Amoxicillin 0.75 g po.
   On hand: Amoxicillin 250 mg per tablet.
   How many tablets would you give? _____

9. Ordered: Valproic acid 15 mg/kg/day.
   Patient's weight: 110 pounds.
   How much valproic acid is given to the patient per day? _____

10. Ordered: Zidovudine 600 mg qd divided into three equal doses.
    On hand: Zidovudine 50 mg/5 mL syrup.
    How many milliliters are given to the patient per day? _____
    How many milliliters are given to the patient in each dose? _____

Dosage Calculations

PRACTICE TEST 4

Name: _____

Define the following terms:

1. tid   =   _____

2. bid   =   _____

3. STAT   =   _____

4. NPO   =   _____

5. gtt   =   _____

6. Ordered: Inderal 20 mg po.
   On hand: Inderal 10 mg per tablet.
   How many tablets would you give? _____

7. Ordered: Amoxicillin 250 mg po.
   On hand: Amoxicillin 125 mg per tablet.
   How many tablets would you give? _____

8. Ordered: Amoxicillin 0.5 g po.
   On hand: Amoxicillin 250 mg per tablet.
   How many tablets would you give? _____

9. Ordered: Rifampin 10 mg/kg/day.
   Patient's weight: 85 kg.
   How much rifampin is given to the patient per day? _____

10. Ordered: Sulfisoxazole 2 g IM.
    On hand: Sulfisoxazole 400 mg/mL.
    How many milliliters of sulfisoxazole are given to the patient? _____

Laboratory and Statistical Calculations

PRACTICE TEST 5

Name: _____

1. Given the following information, calculate the anion gap with and without K^+.
   Sodium   =   132 mmol/L   Anion gap with K^+ =   _____
   Potassium   =   4.5 mmol/L   Anion gap without K^+ =   _____
   Chloride   =   112 mmol/L
   Bicarbonate   =   17 mmol/L

2. Given the following information:
   Sodium   =   165 mmol/L
   Potassium   =   5.9 mmol/L
   Glucose   =   85 mg/dL
   BUN   =   19 mg/dL
   What is the patient's calculated serum osmolality?
   Calculated serum osmolality   =   _____

3. Given the following information:
   Sodium   =   132 mEq/L
   Potassium   =   4.1 mEq/L
   Glucose   =   115 mg/dL
   BUN   =   5 mg/dL
   Serum osmolality =   180 mOsm/kg
   Serum EtOH   =   160 mg/dL
   What is the patient's osmolal gap?   Osmolal gap   =   _____

4. Given the following information, calculate the patient's uncorrected creatinine clearance.
   Serum creatinine   =   1.1 mg/dL   Creatinine clearance   =   _____
   Urine creatinine   =   158 mg/dL
   Time   =   24 hours
   Volume   =   1200 mL

5. A patient's RBC count is 4.5 million/μL, hematocrit = 41%, and hemoglobin = 17 g/dL. Calculate the patient's indices.
   MCV   =   _____   MCH   =   _____
   MCHC =   _____

6. A clean-catch urine specimen obtained from a 25-year-old woman with a possible urinary tract infection is cultured using a 0.01 mL calibrated loop. After appropriate incubation, 350 colonies are counted. What is the patient's CFU/mL count, and is it indicative of a urinary tract infection?
   CFU/mL   =   _____
   Indicative of UTI?   _____ Yes   _____ No   _____ Possible but not probable

7. Given the following set of numbers:
   4, 7, 2, 6, 5, 3, 4, 1
   Calculate the mean.   Mean   =   _____
   Calculate the median.   Median   =   _____
   Calculate the mode.   Mode   =   _____

8. What is the probability that a control result will fall within a 2 standard deviation range?
   Probability   =   _____

9. If the mean for level I glucose control is 100 mg/dL and 1 standard deviation is 5 mg/dL, what is the
   ±1 standard deviation range?   ±1 SD range   =   _____
   ±2 standard deviation range?   ±2 SD range   =   _____
   ±3 standard deviation range?   ±3 SD range   =   _____

10. If analyzer A has a %CV of 3% and analyzer B has a %CV of 5%, which analyzer is more precise?
    _____ Analyzer A   _____ Analyzer B

Laboratory and Statistical Calculations

PRACTICE TEST 6

Name: _____

1. Given the following information, calculate the anion gap with and without K^+.

   Sodium   =   145 mmol/L   Anion gap with K^+ =   _____
   Potassium   =   5.2 mmol/L   Anion gap without K^+ =   _____
   Chloride   =   122 mmol/L
   Bicarbonate   =   12 mmol/L

2. Given the following information:

   Sodium   =   135 mmol/L
   Potassium   =   6.2 mmol/L
   Glucose   =   185 mg/dL
   BUN   =   10 mg/dL

   What is the patient's calculated serum osmolality?
   Calculated serum osmolality   =   _____

3. Given the following information:

   Sodium   =   145 mmol/L
   Potassium   =   4.8 mmol/L
   Glucose   =   125 mg/dL
   BUN   =   18 mg/dL
   Serum osmolality =   192 mOsm/kg
   Serum EtOH   =   180 mg/dL

   What is the patient's osmolal gap?   Osmolal gap   =   _____

4. Given the following information, calculate the patient's uncorrected creatinine clearance.

   Serum creatinine =   2.9 mg/dL   Creatinine clearance   =   _____
   Urine creatinine =   275 mg/dL
   Time   =   24 hours
   Volume   =   1700 mL

5. A patient's RBC count is 3.2 million/μL, hematocrit = 30%, and hemoglobin = 10 g/dL. Calculate the patient's indices.

   MCV   =   _____   MCH   =   _____
   MCHC   =   _____

6. A clean-catch urine specimen obtained from a 2-year-old boy with a possible urinary tract infection is cultured using a 0.01 mL calibrated loop. After appropriate incubation, 70 colonies are counted. What is the patient's CFU/mL count, and is it indicative of a urinary tract infection?

   CFU/mL   =   _____
   Indicative of UTI?   _____ Yes   _____ No   _____ Possible but not probable

7. Given the following set of numbers:
   25, 27, 26, 21, 25, 30, 24, 28
   Calculate the mean.   Mean   = _____
   Calculate the median.   Median = _____
   Calculate the mode.   Mode   = _____

8. What is the probability that a control result will fall within a 1 standard deviation range?
   Probability   =   _____

9. If the mean for level II glucose control is 250 mg/dL and 1 standard deviation is 15 mg/dL, what is the
   ±1 standard deviation range?   ±1 SD range = _____
   ±2 standard deviation range?   ±2 SD range = _____
   ±3 standard deviation range?   ±3 SD range = _____

10. If analyzer A has a %CV of 7% and analyzer B has a %CV of 4%, which analyzer is more precise?
    _____ Analyzer A   _____ Analyzer B

CHAPTER 1

Basic Arithmetic, Rounding Numbers

O B J E C T I V E S

Upon completion of this chapter, the reader should be able to:

1 Perform basic arithmetic calculations, including addition, subtraction, multiplication, and division, with positive and negative numbers.

2 Perform calculations that require multiple steps in the correct order.

3 State the rules for rounding numbers when:
a. The number to be rounded ends in a number less than 5.
b. The number to be rounded ends in a number greater than 5.
c. The number to be rounded ends in 5.

4 Perform calculations including addition, subtraction, multiplication, and division incorporating rules for rounding numbers to achieve the correct result.

INTRODUCTION

Basic Arithmetic

This chapter, as well as Chapters 2 and 3, is designed as a review of basic mathematical concepts. Students already proficient in these concepts may wish to review them briefly and begin at Chapter 4.

Positive and Negative Numbers

A positive number is a number that has a value greater than 0, and a negative number is a number with a value less than 0. Figure 1-1 is a number line that demonstrates this concept. A plus sign (+) is used to identify a positive number, and a negative, or minus, sign (−) is used to identify a negative number. If only positive numbers are used in an equation, the (+) sign is usually omitted.

Addition of Positive Numbers

The sum of two or more positive numbers will also be a positive number (see Fig. 1-2):

$$(+3) + (+15) + (+27) = +45$$

PROBLEMS

What is the sum of +45 and +15?

The sum of +45 and +15 will be a positive number. The sum is obtained by simple addition of the two numbers:

$$(+45) + (+15) = +60$$

Therefore, the sum of +45 and +15 is +60.

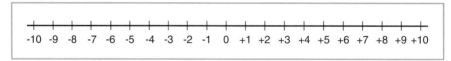

FIGURE 1-1 A number line. (From Doucette, L. J. [1997]. *Basic Mathematics for the Clinical Laboratory* [p. 5]. Philadelphia: W.B. Saunders.)

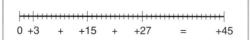

FIGURE 1-2 A number line with three positive numbers added to a positive sum.

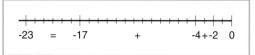

FIGURE 1-3 A number line with three negative numbers added to a negative sum.

What is the sum of +61, +59, +63, +58, +60, +57, and +62?

The sum of this group of numbers will also be a positive number and is obtained by simple addition:

$$(+61) + (+59) + (+63) + (+58) + (+60) + (+57) + (+62) = +420$$

Therefore, the sum of these numbers is $+420$.

Addition of Negative Numbers

The sum of two or more negative numbers will also be a negative number (see Fig. 1-3):

$$(-4) + (-17) + (-2) = -23$$

PROBLEMS

What is the sum of −25 and −15?

The sum of these two negative numbers will also be a negative number and is obtained by simple addition of the two numbers:

$$(-25) + (-15) = -40$$

Therefore, the sum of these two numbers is -40.

What is the sum of −24, −32, −21, −31?

The sum of this group of numbers is determined by simple addition:

$$(-24) + (-32) + (-21) + (-31) = -108$$

Therefore, the sum of this group of numbers is -108.

Addition of Both Positive and Negative Numbers

The sum of an addition of both positive and negative numbers will be the sign of the larger number involved in the addition. If you think of the numbers on the number line as players in a "tug-of-war" game, then the larger number will be able to "pull" the smaller number in the direction of the sign of the larger number.

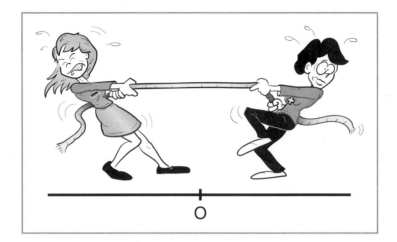

That is, if the larger number is positive, then the smaller number is pulled in the positive direction. When a negative number is added to a positive number, in reality it is actually *subtracted from* the positive number. For example, what is the sum of −21 and +15?

Because the larger number is a negative number, the sum will have a negative number. By convention, when placing the numbers in correct order to perform the calculation, the positive number is listed first, followed by the negative number. The negative number is actually subtracted from the positive number to arrive at the sum.

+15 −21 = −6

The sum of these two numbers is −6, a negative number.

PROBLEMS

What is the sum of −54 and +25?

When presented with an equation that contains both positive and negative numbers, first arrange the numbers in the equation so that the positive number(s) are listed first, followed by the negative number(s):

(+25) + (−54)

Then, solve the equation:

(+25) + (−54) = X
25 − 54 = −29

In this equation, the negative number was larger than the positive number, causing the sum to be a negative number. Remember, think of the numbers as being engaged in a tug of war. The sign of the larger number will tug the equation in its direction and determine the sign of the final quotient. In this example, since −54 is larger than +25, the final quotient of 29 is a negative number, i.e., −29.

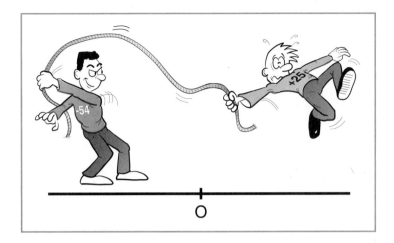

What is the sum of −21, +54, +12, −32, −5, +10?

First, organize the numbers so that all of the positive numbers are listed first, followed by the negative numbers. The numbers do not have to be listed in rank order, i.e., smallest to largest.

+12, +10, +54, −21, −32, −5

Next, determine the sum of the positive numbers:

(+12) + (+10) + (+54) = +76

Then, determine the sum of the negative numbers:

(−21) + (−32) + (−5) = −58

Last, set up the final equation of the sums of both the positive and negative groups of numbers, listing the positive number first:

(+76) + (−58) = X

Now solve for X, using the rules for addition of both positive and negative numbers: (+76) + (−58) = X

76 − 58 = X
18 = X

Therefore, the sum of this group of mixed positive and negative numbers is +18.

Subtraction of Two or More Positive Numbers

If the answer is greater than 0, it remains a positive number. However, if a larger positive number is subtracted from a smaller positive number, the answer will have a value less than 0 and will be a negative number. For example:

25 − 35 = −10

PROBLEMS

What is the answer to the following equation: 43 − 13 = x?

This equation can be solved using simple arithmetic. Subtract 13 from 43:

$$43 - 13 = 30$$

The answer, 30, is also a positive number because its value remains above 0.

Solve the following equation: 12 − 20 = x.

This equation can also be solved using simple arithmetic. However, because 20 is larger than 12, the final answer, −8, will be a negative number.

$$12 - 20 = -8$$

Subtraction of Two or More Negative Numbers

When two negative numbers are subtracted from each other, the answer remains negative as long as it is less than 0. However, similar to working with positive numbers, if a larger negative number is subtracted from a smaller negative number, the answer will have a value greater than 0 and will be a positive number. This is because when a negative number is subtracted from a positive or negative number it is actually *added to* the positive or negative number because of the following rule:

Two negatives become a positive.

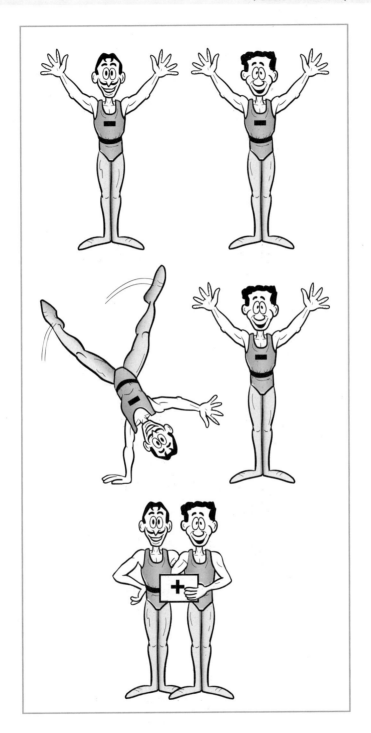

Whether the final result is a positive or negative number depends on how much pull there is on the number line by the numbers in the equation.

PROBLEMS

Solve the following equation: $(-12) - (-3) = X$.

In this equation, because -3 is being subtracted from -12, the double negatives convert into a positive (+) sign for the number 3.

$(-12) + (3) = X$

This equation can be rearranged with the positive number listed first:

$3 - 12 = X$
$X = -9$

The final answer is still a negative number because the -3 did not have enough pull to make the final result a positive number.

Solve the following equation: $(-5) - (-7) = X$.

Again, because two negatives make a positive, the sign associated with the number 7 is changed to a positive.

$(-5) + (7) = X$

Again, the equation can be rearranged so that the positive number is listed first:

$7 - 5 = X$
$2 = X$

In this case, the final result is a positive number because the number 7 had enough pull to shift the final result over the 0 value in the number line.

Multiplication or Division of Two or More Positive Numbers

When two or more positive numbers are multiplied or divided, the result will be a *positive* number.

PROBLEMS

Solve the following equation: $(9) \times (3) = X$.

This equation of two positive numbers can be solved using simple multiplication:

$9 \times 3 = 27$

The product, 27, is also a positive number.

Solve the following equation: $(60) \div (2) = X$.

This equation of two positive numbers can be solved by simple division:

$$60 \div 2 = 30$$

The result, 30, is also a positive number.

Multiplication or Division of Two or More Negative Numbers

When two or more negative numbers are multiplied or divided, the result will be a *positive* number.

PROBLEM

Solve the following equation: $(-12) \times (-3) = X$.

This equation can be solved by simple multiplication. Because two negatives make a positive, the final result will be a positive number:

$$(-12) \times (-3) = 36$$

Therefore, the result, 36, is a positive number.

Multiplication or Division of Negative and Positive Numbers

The result obtained when two or more negative numbers are multiplied or divided together will be a *positive* number. By contrast, when positive and negative numbers are multiplied or divided together, the result will be a *negative* number.

PROBLEMS

Solve the following equation: $(5) \times (-4) = X$.

This equation can be solved using simple multiplication. However, because one of the numbers involved in the equation is negative, the final result will also be a negative number.

$$(5) \times (-4) = -20$$

The result, −20, is a negative number.

Solve the following equation: $(-24) \div (6) = X$.

This equation can be solved by simple division; however, remember that the final result will be a *negative* number.

$$(-24) \div (6) = -4$$

Therefore, the result of this equation is −4.

Order of Calculations

When an equation contains numbers within parentheses, the calculation within the parentheses is performed first. For example, the equation 23 + (43 × 2) is solved by first performing the calculation within the parentheses. The equation then becomes 23 + 86, a simple addition problem.

PROBLEM

Solve the following equation: 52 − (75 ÷ 15) = X.

First, solve the equation within the parentheses.

75 ÷ 15 = 5

Next, substitute the answer to the equation, 5, into the original equation:

52 − 5 = X

Finally, using simple subtraction, solve for X:

52 − 5 = 47

Thus, the answer to the equation 52 − (75 ÷ 15) is 47.

Rounding Numbers

In health care, the preciseness of a measurement is determined by using the rules that guide the use of significant figures and rounding numbers. Significant figures will be discussed in detail in Chapter 2. *Rounding off* is the process of removing excess digits from a number in order for that number to have its correct quantity of significant figures. For example, when using a calculator, the result shown on the display may contain many digits, far more than are necessary for the equation solved. By using the rules for rounding numbers, the digits can be reduced to the correct significant quantity.

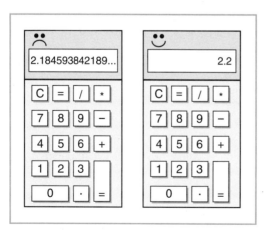

Rules for Rounding Numbers

If the First Digit to Be Dropped Is Less Than 5

If the first digit to be dropped is less than 5, then the last remaining digit stays the same.

PROBLEMS

Round the number 13.793 from five to four significant figures.

Since the digit to be dropped is less than 5, the last remaining digit, 9, stays the same and the number becomes 13.79.

Round the number 7.44 from three to two significant figures.

Since the digit to be dropped is less than 5, the last remaining digit, 4, stays the same and the number becomes 7.4.

If the First Digit to Be Dropped Is Greater Than 5

If the first digit to be dropped is greater than 5, then the last remaining digit is rounded to the next highest digit.

PROBLEMS

Round the number 8.67 from three to two significant figures.

The digit 7 is dropped, and since it is higher than 5, the digit 6 is rounded to 7. Thus the number becomes 8.7.

Round the number 45.189 from five to four significant figures.

The digit 9 is dropped, and since it is higher than 5, the digit 8 is rounded to 9. Thus the number becomes 45.19.

If the First Digit to Be Dropped Is the Number 5

If the first digit to be dropped is the number 5, the last remaining digit is rounded to the next higher number if it is an *odd* number. If the last remaining digit is an *even* number, then it is unchanged.

PROBLEMS

Round the number 2.35 from three to two significant figures.

Since the last digit is 5 and the next digit is an odd number, 3, the odd number is rounded to the next even number. Thus the final number becomes 2.4.

Round the number 1.75 from three to two significant figures.

Since the last digit is 5 and the next digit is an odd number, 7, the odd number is rounded to the next even number. Thus the final number becomes 1.8.

Round the number 39265 from five to four significant figures.

The 5 is dropped, but since the next digit, 6, is an even number, it is unchanged. Thus the number becomes 3926, not 3927.

Round the number 4.825 from four to three significant figures.

Since the last digit is 5 and the next digit is an even number, 2, the even number is unchanged. Thus the final number becomes 4.82.

EXAMPLE PROBLEMS

This section is designed to be useful to both the student and the health care practitioner. Students can use the example problems in order to master the material. The health care practitioner can use these problems as templates for solving calculations. Find an example problem similar to the problem that you need to solve and substitute into the equation the numbers appropriate to your calculation.

1. **Q** **What is the sum of (+13) + (+80)?**

   A The sum of two positive numbers will be a positive number. The sum is calculated using simple addition: 13 + 80 = 93. Therefore, the sum is +93.

2. **Q** **What is the sum of (+450) + (+200)?**

   A The sum will be a positive number and is calculated using simple addition: 450 + 200 = +650.

3. **Q** **What is the sum of (−31) + (−4)?**

   A The sum of two or more negative numbers will be a negative number and is calculated using simple addition without initial regard for the signs of the numbers: 31 + 4 = 35. The sum, 35, is then given a negative sign, −35.

4. **Q** **What is the sum of the following group of numbers: −40, −10, −50?**

   A The sum of a group of negative numbers is also a negative number and can be calculated using simple addition: (−40) + (−10) + (−50) = −100.

5. **Q** **What is the sum of −15 and +10?**

   A The sign of the sum of an equation with both negative and positive numbers depends on which number is larger and its associated sign. Usually, the positive number in the equation is listed first and the negative number is actually subtracted from the positive number. Therefore, the equation is rewritten as $10 - 15 = ?$ and solved using simple subtraction: $10 - 15 = -5$. The sum is a negative number because the negative number in this equation, −15, is larger than the positive number, 10, and pulls the sum over the number line to be a negative number.

6. **Q** **What is the sum of −4 and +12?**

   A An equation containing both positive and negative numbers is rewritten so that the positive number appears first: $12 - 4 = ?$ and is solved by simple subtraction: $12 - 4 = 8$. The sum, 8, is a positive number because it was not pulled across the number line by the −4.

7. **Q** **What is the sum of the following group of numbers: −5, −10, +3, +8, −4?**

   A First, rewrite the equation to place the positive numbers first, followed by the negative numbers: $(+3) + (+8) + (-5) + (-10) + (-4) = ?$ Next, determine the sum of the positive numbers: $3 + 8 + 5 = 16$. Then, determine the sum of the negative numbers: $(-10) + (-4) = (-14)$. Finally, set up the equation using the sums of the positive and negative numbers: $16 - 14 = 2$. Therefore, the sum of this group of numbers is 2.

8. **Q** **What is the answer to the following equation: $18 - 8 = ?$**

   A This is solved using simple arithmetic: $18 - 8 = 10$.

9. **Q** **What is the answer to the following equation: $73 - 27 = ?$**

   A The answer can be determined by simple subtraction: $73 - 27 = 46$.

10. **Q** **What is the answer to the following equation: $(-35) - (-20) = ?$**

    A Using the rule that two negatives become a positive, the equation can be rewritten as follows: $-35 + 20 = ?$ Then the equation can be rewritten with the positive number listed first: $20 - 35 = ?$ Finally, the equation can be solved: $20 - 35 = -15$.

11. **Q** **What is the answer to the following equation: $(-4) - (-6) = ?$**

    A First, rewrite the equation as $-4 + 6 = ?$ Then, rewrite the equation listing the positive 6 first: $6 - 4 = ?$ Last, solve the equation: $6 - 4 = 2$.

12. **Q** What is the answer to the following equation: (3) × (25) = ?

   A Using simple multiplication to solve this problem yields the following: 3 × 25 = 75.

13. **Q** Solve the following equation: (45) × (5) = ?

   A This problem can be solved using simple arithmetic: 45 × 5 = 225.

14. **Q** Solve the following equation: 15 ÷ 3 = ?

   A This problem can be solved using simple division: 15 ÷ 3 = 5.

15. **Q** Solve the following equation: 70 ÷ 10 = ?

   A This problem can be solved using simple division: 70 ÷ 10 = 7.

16. **Q** Solve the following equation: (−3) × (−4) = ?

   A This problem can also be solved using simple arithmetic. However, because of the rule that two negatives make a positive, the answer will be a positive number: (−3) × (−4) = 12.

17. **Q** Solve the following equation: (−11) × (−3) = ?

   A The answer to the problem is +33.

18. **Q** Solve the following equation: (−14) ÷ (−7) = ?

   A The answer to the problem is +2.

19. **Q** Solve the following equation: (6) × (−3) = ?

   A This problem can be solved using simple multiplication. However, because one of the numbers in the equation is negative, the final result will also be a negative number: (6) × (−3) = − 18.

20. **Q** Solve the following equation: (−7) × (4) = ?

   A The answer to the problem is −28.

21. **Q** Solve the following equation: (−12) ÷ (3) = ?

   A Again, the final result will be a negative number: (−12) ÷ (3) = −4.

22. **Q** If 8.813 is to be rounded to three significant figures, what will the final number be?

   A The final number will be 8.81. The 3 would be dropped and the 1 would remain unchanged since 3 is less than 5.

23. **Q** If 94.82 is rounded to three significant figures, what will the final number be?

   A The final number will be 94.8. The 2 will be dropped, and since it is less than 5, the 8 remains unchanged.

24. **Q** If 5.46 is rounded to two significant figures, what will the final number be?

A 5.46 will be rounded to 5.5. The 6 is dropped, and since 6 is more than 5, the 4 is changed to 5.

25. **Q** **The number 9.24 must be rounded to two significant figures. What will the final number be?**

A The final number will be 9.2. The 4 is dropped, and the 2 is rounded to 3.

26. **Q** **If the number 6.97 is rounded to two significant figures, what will the number be?**

A 6.97 will be rounded to 7.0. The 7 will be dropped and the 9 rounded to 10. This changes the 6 to 7.

27. **Q** **If the number 7.35 is rounded to two significant figures, what will the final number be?**

A 7.35 will be rounded to 7.4. Remember that when the digit to be dropped is 5, the next digit is rounded up if it is an odd number but unchanged if it is an even number.

28. **Q** **If the number 0.4825 is rounded to three significant figures, what will the number be?**

A 0.4825 will become 0.482. The 5 is dropped since only three, not four, significant numbers are needed. However, since the next digit is an even number, it remains unchanged.

Practice Problems

Solve the following practice problems to further master the material. All answers and explanations to some problems can be found in a separate section at the back of the book.

Solve the following problems:

1. $5 + 27$ = ?
2. $13 + 6$ = ?
3. $21 + 16$ = ?
4. $10 + 4$ = ?
5. $(-13) + (-5)$ = ?
6. $(-2) + (-52)$ = ?
7. $(-61) + (-30)$ = ?
8. $(-75) + (+5)$ = ?
9. $(-22) + (+11)$ = ?
10. $(-10) + (-41) + (+16) + (+8)$ = ?

11. $(+21) + (+64) + (-71) + (-14)$ = ?
12. $80 - 20$ = ?
13. $12 - 5$ = ?
14. $(-15) - (-5)$ = ?
15. $(-73) - (-17)$ = ?
16. $(-41) - (-45)$ = ?
17. 52×3 = ?
18. 14×6 = ?
19. 22×3 = ?
20. $35 \div 5$ = ?
21. $40 \div 4$ = ?
22. $(-15) \div (-3)$ = ?
23. $(-33) \div (-3)$ = ?
24. $(-42) \div (+2)$ = ?
25. $(+14) \div (-7)$ = ?

Round the following numbers to three significant figures.

26. 0.6293
27. 12.74
28. 4.987
29. 6.669
30. 5.558
31. 3.635
32. 2.825

Significant Figures and Scientific Notation

INTRODUCTION

Significant Figures

Significant figures are used in science to determine the precision of measurements. If you are measuring the height of a patient, you have to know how precise the measurement should be. There is an implied degree of uncertainty in the precision of any measurement. If an instrument is found to be 33.4 inches long using a ruler that is precise only to the tenths, then the actual measurement could be anywhere between 33.400 and 33.459 inches long. By using significant figures, the degree of implied uncertainty of measurements can be established.

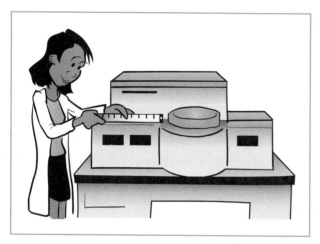

In general, the exactness of a group of measurements depends on the *least* exact measurement. For example, if you were given the volumes of 10.0 mL, 15.85 mL, and 7.775 mL for three different solutions that needed to be added together, the *sum* of these three solutions would not be 33.625 but rather 33.6. This is because, of the three measurements taken, 10.0 mL has the fewest number of significant figures. You do not know if 10.05 mL instead of 10.0 mL was actually measured. The 10.0 mL measurement is precise only to the first decimal place. Because this measurement is limited in its precision, all of the other measurements must be limited in their precision as well.

The precision of a number can be noted in different ways. A less popular method is to place a bar over the least significant digit in a number. For example, in the number 487$\overline{4}$, the number is exact only to 4870 since the 4 has a bar over it.

Another method is to place a decimal point at the end of the number to emphasize its precision. If directions for an intravenous (IV) solution called for 1250. mL of physiologic saline, then any measurement between 1250.10 and 1250.49 mL of saline would be within the boundaries of the precision of the number 1250. In this example, the directions are only precise enough so that the measurement must be between 1250. and 1250.5 mL.

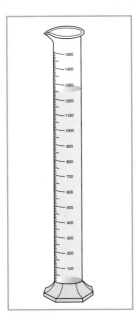

However, in other situations, the measurements may need to be much more precise. In many areas of the clinical laboratory, measurements of solids such as salts are commonly taken to the second or third decimal place. Liquids may be measured by using a volumetric flask or by weighing. In either case, it is common to determine the precision of the measurement by using a decimal point and digits to the right of the decimal point. For example, if 5.75 g of calcium carbonate needed to be weighed, then the technologist would measure to the hundredth of a gram. On the other hand, if a doctor ordered a glucose test on a diabetic patient, the amount of glucose to be measured would be precise only to the gram and would be reported only in whole numbers. Other laboratory values, such as pH, are reported to the hundredth, i.e., a pH of 7.35. instead of a whole number, i.e., 7.

A third common way to express the precision of a number is to use scientific notation. For example, 1000. could be written as 10×10^2 or 164,328 could be written as 16.4328×10^4. A number less than 1, such as 0.00365, could be written as 3.65×10^{-3}. In most scientific measurements, scientific notation is used most often because it is the most error-free method to denote precision.

Working with Significant Figures

Significant Figures and 0s

There are some rules to remember when using numbers that contain 0s when working with significant figures.

Numbers That Contain 0s Internally
When a number contains a 0 or 0s internally, the 0 or 0s are considered to be significant to that number and are never dropped out of the number.

PROBLEMS

How many significant figures are within the number 2,580,593.?

The number 2,580,593. has seven significant figures. The 0 within the number is a significant number because it designates the thousandth's position. The decimal point after the last 3 signifies that the 3 in the one's position is the least significant number and that this number is precise to the nearest whole number.

How many significant figures are within the number 9587.0083?

The number 9587.0083 has eight significant figures. The two 0s to the right of the decimal point are significant because they are within the entire number.

How many significant figures are within the number 9107.022?

The number 9107.022 has seven significant figures. Both 0s are significant because they are within the entire number.

Numbers That Contain 0s at the End of the Number

When a number contains a 0 or 0s at the end of the number, or to the right of the decimal place, the 0 or 0s are considered to be significant.

PROBLEMS

How many significant figures are within the number 34,500.?

The number 34,500. has five significant figures. It can also easily be rewritten using scientific notation as 3.45×10^4, and in this form it has only three significant figures.

How many significant figures are within the number 86,510.0?

The number 86,510.0 has six significant figures. It also can easily be rewritten using scientific notation as 8.651×10^4, and in this form it has only four significant figures.

How many significant figures are within the number 781.0?

The number 781.0 has four significant figures. It also can easily be rewritten using scientific notation as 7.81×10^2 and would have three significant figures.

Numbers Less Than 1 That Contain 0s to the Right of the Decimal Point

When a number is less than 1, any 0 that is between the decimal point and the first digit within the number is *not* considered to be significant.

PROBLEMS

How many significant figures are within the number 0.0931?

The number 0.0931 has three significant figures, not four, and, using scientific notation, can be rewritten as 9.31×10^{-2}.

How many significant figures are within the number 0.00314?

The number 0.00314 has three significant figures, not five, and, using scientific notation, can be rewritten as 3.14×10^{-3}.

How many significant figures are within the number 0.000812?

The number 0.000812 has three significant figures, not six, and, using scientific notation, can be rewritten as 8.12×10^{-4}.

Significant Figures in Addition and Subtraction

There are rules when working with significant figures and performing calculations. For calculations involving addition or subtraction, the sum or product of a group of numbers is no more precise than the least precise number in the group of numbers that were added or subtracted. The final product of an addition or subtraction problem can have as many digits to the right of the decimal point as the least precise number involved in the problem.

PROBLEMS

What is the sum of these numbers?

```
   10.5
   14.386
 + 12.65
   37.536 = 37.5
```

The answer can be precise only to the one-tenth position since 10.5 is precise only to five-tenths.

What is the sum of these numbers?

```
   465.2
     7.436
 +  12.51
   485.146 = 485.1
```

485.146 becomes 485.1 because the number 465.2 is precise only to the one-tenth position and the final sum cannot be more precise than the least precise number in the problem.

What is the difference between these numbers?

$$8.53$$
$$-\ \underline{4.1}$$
$$4.43 = 4.4$$

4.43 becomes 4.4 because it can have only two significant figures since 4.1 is precise only to the nearest one-tenth.

What is the difference between these numbers?

$$10.467$$
$$-\ \underline{2.45}$$
$$8.017 = 8.02$$

The difference is 8.02, not 8.017, since 2.45 is precise only to the one-one-hundredth position, not the one-one-thousandth position.

Significant Figures in Multiplication and Division

When performing multiplication and division calculations, the final product cannot contain more significant figures than the number in the calculation with the fewest number of significant figures.

PROBLEMS

What is the answer to this problem?

$$5.251$$
$$\times\ \underline{2.74}$$
$$14.38774 = 14.4$$

The final answer is 14.4 because 2.74 with three significant figures is the limiting number.

What is the answer to this problem?

$$0.532$$
$$\times\ \underline{0.047}$$
$$0.025 = 0.025$$

The final answer does not need to be changed since it has the same number of significant figures, two, as the limiting number, 0.047.

What is the answer to this problem?

$$25.94 \div 8.1 = 3.20$$
$$3.20 = 3.2$$

The answer is 3.2, not 3.20, because 8.1 has the fewest number of significant figures.

What is the answer to this problem?

0.92 ÷ 0.45 = 2.0

The answer, 2.0, does not change, as it has the correct amount of significant figures.

Exponents and Scientific Notation

In mathematics, multiplication is used because it is faster than simple addition when performing multiple addition problems. For example, $5 \times 8 = 40$. The same answer could be found by adding 5 eight times: $5 + 5 + 5 + 5 + 5 + 5 + 5 + 5 = 40$. *Exponents* are a further way to simplify complex multiplication problems.

Exponents are written as x^a where x is called the *base* and a is the *exponent*. The base is the number that is to be multiplied by itself, and the exponent determines how many times it will be multiplied.

For example, 2^4 is equal to $2 \times 2 \times 2 \times 2$ or 16. In complicated calculations involving many exponents, it is easy to see how the use of exponents can reduce the chance of making errors in performing the arithmetic of the calculation.

In science, *scientific notation* is often used in calculations to avoid errors in very large or very small numbers. In scientific notation, a number is written in such a way that it is larger than 1 but less than 10 and an integral power of 10. For example, the number 23600000.0 can be expressed as 2.36×10^7.

There are some simple rules for using scientific notation. If these rules are learned and understood, errors in calculations using scientific notation will be reduced.

Rule 1

Exponents used in scientific notation can be positive or negative numbers. Exponents that are negative usually indicate a number that is less than 1. A negative sign is placed to the left of the exponent to indicate that it is a negative exponent. Exponents that are positive generally do not have any sign associated with them. It is assumed that if a negative sign is not present, the exponent is positive.

PROBLEM

What is the numerical value of the following positive exponents?

2×10^3

7×10^2

Remember that in scientific notation, the number is written to be between 1 and 10, with a power of 10.

$2 \times 10^3 = (2) \times (10)(10)(10) = 2 \times 1000 = 2000$

$7 \times 10^2 = (7) \times (10)(10) = 7 \times 100 = 700$

Numbers with negative exponents are expressed with the following formula:

$$b^{-a} = \frac{1}{b^a}$$

PROBLEM

What is the numerical value of the negative exponent 4×10^{-5}?

In this example, from the equation for negative exponents, $b = 10$ and $a = -5$.

$$4 \times 10^{-5} = 4 \times \frac{1}{10^5}$$

$$4 \times \frac{1}{10^5} = 4 \times \frac{1}{100000} = 0.00004$$

Notice that with scientific notation the final product could easily be obtained by simply moving the decimal point to the left for a negative exponent and to the right for a positive exponent the number of times indicated by the exponent number itself. In the example above, 2×10^3 was shown to be equal to 2000. Instead of multiplying 10 by itself three times, simply use 2.0 as the starting point and move the decimal to the right three places.

2.0	2 0 .0	2 0 0 .0	2 0 0 0 .0
Base number	1 decimal place	2 decimal places	3 decimal places

For a negative exponent, the decimal place is moved to the left. Using 4×10^{-5} from the second example, the decimal point is moved five places to the left.

4.0	0 . 4	0 .0 4	0 .0 0 4	0 .0 0 0 4	0 .0 0 0 0 4
Base number	1 decimal place	2 decimal places	3 decimal places	4 decimal places	5 decimal places

TABLE 2-1   Exponents, Their Values, and Examples

Exponent	Number and Exp.	Value	Example
$10^0 = 1$	$a \times 10^0$	a	$5 \times 10^0 = 5$
$10^1 = 10$	$a \times 10^1$	$a \times 10$	$5 \times 10^1 = 50$
$10^2 = 100$	$a \times 10^2$	$a \times 100$	$5 \times 10^2 = 500$
$10^3 = 1000$	$a \times 10^3$	$a \times 1000$	$5 \times 10^3 = 5000$
$10^6 = 1,000,000$	$a \times 10^6$	$a \times 1,000,000$	$5 \times 10^6 = 5,000,000$
$10^9 = 1,000,000,000$	$a \times 10^9$	$a \times 1,000,000,000$	$5 \times 10^9 = 5,000,000,000$
$10^{-1} = 0.1$	$a \times 10^{-1}$	$a \times 0.1$	$5 \times 10^{-1} = 0.5$
$10^{-2} = 0.01$	$a \times 10^{-2}$	$a \times 0.01$	$5 \times 10^{-2} = 0.05$
$10^{-3} = 0.001$	$a \times 10^{-3}$	$a \times 0.001$	$5 \times 10^{-3} = 0.005$
$10^{-6} = 0.000001$	$a \times 10^{-6}$	$a \times 0.000001$	$5 \times 10^{-6} = 0.000005$
$10^{-9} = 0.000000001$	$a \times 10^{-9}$	$a \times 0.000000001$	$5 \times 10^{-9} = 0.000000005$

Rule 2

Any number greater than 0 that has an exponent raised to the 0 power has a value of 1. Using scientific notation, the power of 10 would have an exponent of 0. This is expressed mathematically as:

$$b \times 10^0 = b \times 1 = b$$

A good understanding of how exponents function in scientific notation may help to show why the power of 10 raised to the 0 power has a value of 1. The exponent indicates how many times 10 must be multiplied by itself. The 0 exponent simply means that the power of 10 in scientific notation is to be used 0 times or not to be used at all. The number associated with the power of 10 remains the same, i.e., multiplied by 1. Table 2-1 demonstrates commonly used powers of 10 and their value.

PROBLEMS

What is 5.8×10^0?

This problem can be solved two different ways: From Table 2-1, $10^0 = 1$. Substituting this equivalent value into the equation yields 5.8×1, which equals 5.8. From Table 2-1, $a \times 10^0 = a$, or, using the example, $5 \times 10^0 = 5$. By substituting the numbers in the problem into the equation, then, $5.8 \times 10^0 = 5.8$.

What is 9.2×10^3?

Using Table 2-1, $10^3 = 1000$. Substituting this equivalent value into the equation yields 9.2×1000, which equals 9200. From Table 2-1, $a \times 10^3 = a \times 1000$, or, using the example, $5 \times 10^3 = 5000$. By substituting the numbers in the problem into the equation, then, $9.2 \times 10^3 = 9200$.

Rule 3

When multiplying two numbers using scientific notation, the numbers themselves are multiplied but the exponents are added. This rule can be expressed as follows:

$$[(b \times 10^a)(c \times 10^d)] = (bc)^{a+d}$$

PROBLEM

Multiply 6.5×10^2 by 3.9×10^3.

Using rule 2, the following equation is derived:

$$[(6.5 \times 10^2)(3.9 \times 10^3)] = [(6.5)(3.9)]10^{2+3} = 25 \times 10^5 \text{ or } 2.5 \times 10^6$$

This equation can be verified by using simple arithmetic:

$6.5 \times 10^2 = 650$
$3.9 \times 10^3 = 3900$
$650 \times 3900 = 2{,}535{,}000$

The difference between 2,535,000 and 2.5×10^6 is due to rules of calculation involving significant figures. The number 2,535,000 is rounded to two significant figures.

Rule 4

When a number in scientific notation is multiplied by an exponent, the base number is multiplied by itself the number of times expressed by the exponent. The power of 10 exponent is multiplied by the exponent. This is expressed mathematically as:

$$(a \times 10^b)^c = a^c \times 10^{bc}$$

a^c is equal to a multiplied by itself c times. This is expressed mathematically as:

$$a^c = a \times a \times a \ldots \quad (c \text{ times})$$

Thus,

$$(2.5 \times 10^2)^2 = 2.5^2 \times 10^{2 \times 2} = (2.5 \times 2.5) \times (10 \times 10 \times 10 \times 10) = 6.2 \times 10^4$$

Rule 5

In a division calculation involving numbers in scientific notation, the exponent in the denominator is subtracted from the exponent in the numerator of the equation. This rule is expressed mathematically as:

$$\frac{a \times 10^b}{c \times 10^d} = \frac{a \times 10^{b-d}}{c}$$

PROBLEM

Divide 7.95 × 10³ by 2.5 × 10².

Using the formula from rule 5:

$$\frac{7.95 \times 10^3}{2.5 \times 10^2} = \frac{7.95}{2.5} \times 10^{3-2} = 3.2 \times 10^1$$

This answer can be confirmed by simple arithmetic:

$$7.95 \times 10^3 = 7950$$
$$2.5 \times 10^2 = 250$$
$$\frac{7950}{250} = 31.8 = 3.2 \times 10^1$$

All calculations performed using scientific notation should arrive at the same answer that could be obtained by the slower simple arithmetic method. It is a good idea to check your answers while becoming familiar with scientific notation to make sure that mistakes are not made.

Rule 6

A different but comparable way of expressing a division problem is the rule that in a division problem, the exponent in the numerator can be subtracted from the exponent in the denominator, but only when the division equation of the exponents is inverted. This is expressed mathematically as:

$$\frac{a \times 10^b}{c \times 10^d} = \frac{a}{c} \times \frac{1}{10^{d-b}}$$

The calculation from the previous problem will be used to demonstrate rule 6. Using the formula from rule 6:

$$\frac{7.95 \times 10^3}{2.5 \times 10^2} = \frac{7.95}{2.5} \times \frac{1}{10^{2-3}} = 3.2 \times \frac{1}{10^{-1}}$$

$$3.2 \times \frac{1}{10^{-1}} = 3.2 \times 10^1$$

When a negative exponent is in the denominator of an equation, it becomes positive when inverted to the numerator. This is why $1/10^{-1}$ became a positive 10^1.

Rule 7

When performing addition and subtraction using scientific notation, it is easy to make arithmetic errors. This is because, when performing addition and subtraction, the power of 10 exponents used for scientific notation do not follow the same rules as for multiplication and division. The best way to proceed is to first convert all the numbers in the calculation to their original nonscientific notation form and then perform the addition or subtraction. When using a calculator to perform addition or subtraction involving scientific notation, the EXP function is used. The calculator will convert the numbers to their nonexponent form when performing the calculation.

PROBLEMS

Add $7.23 \times 10^4 + 9.2 \times 10^2$.

If we try to solve this problem manually using the same exponent rule as for multiplication, then the equation that will be derived is:

$(7.23 + 9.2) \times 10^6$

Will this equation result in the correct answer? No! Logic tells us that this equation cannot result in the correct answer.

If, however, we first convert each number expressed in scientific notation back to its simpler form and then perform the addition, we arrive at

$72{,}300 + 920 = 73{,}220$ or 7.3×10^4

Subtract 1.3×10^2 from 8.5×10^3.

In subtraction, there is no easy way to perform the calculation without a good chance of making errors except by first converting all terms into their simpler forms if the subtraction is performed manually or by using the EXP function of a calculator.

$8500 - 130 = 8370$ or 8.4×10^3

Up to this point, all of the examples have used positive exponents. The same rules apply when working with negative exponents. A common mistake when performing calculations involving negative exponents is to forget that when a negative number is subtracted from a positive number, it is actually *added to* the positive number because of the following rule presented in Chapter 1:

Two negatives become a positive.

PROBLEM

Divide 4.0×10^{-2} by 6.0×10^{-3}.

Using the rules of division with exponents, the following equation is derived:

$$\frac{4.0 \times 10^{-2}}{6.0 \times 10^{-3}} = \frac{4}{6} \times 10^{-2-(-3)} =$$

$$0.66 \times 10^1 = 6.6$$

OR

$$\frac{4.0 \times 10^{-2}}{6.0 \times 10^{-3}} = \frac{4}{6} \times \frac{1}{10^{-3-(-2)}} =$$

$$0.66 \times 10^1 = 6.6$$

When −3 is subtracted from −2, it is actually *added to* −2 and so becomes a positive number (+1).

To confirm these answers, convert all numbers to their original nonscientific notation form:

$$4.0 \times 10^{-2} = 0.04$$
$$6.0 \times 10^{-3} = 0.006$$
$$\frac{0.04}{0.006} = 6.6$$

EXAMPLE PROBLEMS

This section is designed to be useful to both the student and the health care practitioner. Students can use the example problems in order to master the material. The health care practitioner can use these problems as templates for solving calculations. Find an example problem similar to the problem that you need to solve and substitute into the equation the numbers appropriate to your calculation.

1. **Q** **The number 8.93 has how many significant figures?**
   A This number has three significant figures and is precise to the one-one-hundredth place.

2. **Q** **The number 64.077 has how many significant figures?**
   A This number has five significant figures and is precise to the one-one-thousandth place.

3. **Q** **How many significant figures are contained in the number 7500.?**
   A This number contains four significant figures. The 0s are significant because they are followed by a period. Remember that a period at the end of a number may also be used to denote significant figures.

4. **Q** **How many significant figures are contained in the number 0.00912?**
   A This number has three significant figures. Remember that 0s that fall before or after a decimal point but precede any numbers are not significant.

5. **Q** How many significant figures are contained in the number 0.02081?

   A This number has four significant figures. The 0s on either side of the decimal point are *not* significant, whereas the zero *within* the number *is* significant.

6. **Q** How many significant figures are contained in the number 5480.00?

   A This number contains six significant figures. The 0s before and after the decimal point are significant because they describe the preciseness of the number.

7. **Q** The sum of 25.4 + 32.9 has how many significant figures?

   A The sum, 58.3, has three significant figures.

8. **Q** The sum of 25.29 + 8.4 has how many significant figures?

   A The sum, 33.7, has three significant figures. Remember that the sum of a group of numbers cannot be more precise than the least precise number in the problem.

9. **Q** 45.2 − 2.6 results in an answer with how many significant figures?

   A The answer, 42.6, contains three significant figures.

10. **Q** The product of 2.55 × 8.97 contains how many significant figures?

    A The product, 22.9, contains three significant figures. Remember that in multiplication, the final product cannot contain more significant figures than the least precise number in the problem.

11. **Q** How many significant figures does the product of 0.123 × 0.871 contain?

    A The product, 0.107, contains three significant figures.

12. **Q** 856.1 ÷ 9.2 results in an answer with how many significant figures?

    A The answer, 93, contains two significant figures. You may have calculated the answer to be 93.05. Remember, in division, the final answer cannot contain more significant figures than the least significant number in the problem. Since 9.2 contains two significant figures, the final answer is limited to two significant figures.

13. **Q** How many significant figures are contained in the answer to 2.37 ÷ 0.25?

    A The answer, 9.5, contains two significant figures.

14. **Q** **Express 240,000,000.00 in exponent form.**
    A 240,000,000.00 is equal to 2.4×10^8.

15. **Q** **Express 0.000435 in exponent form.**
    A 0.000435 is equal to 4.35×10^{-4}.

16. **Q** **Multiply 9.4×10^4 by 8.2×10^2.**
    A The rule for multiplication with scientific notation states that when multiplying two or more numbers with exponents, the numbers themselves are multiplied but the exponents are added. Therefore, the equation would be $[(9.4)(8.2)]^{4+2} = 7.7 \times 10^7$.

17. **Q** **Multiply 6.73×10^2 by 8.2×10^3.**
    A $[(6.73)(8.2)]^{2+3} = 55.2 \times 10^5$, which becomes 5.5×10^6.

18. **Q** **What is 3.1×10^2 squared?**
    A When multiplying a number in scientific notation by an exponent, the base number is multiplied by itself the number of times expressed by the exponent's value, while the exponent associated with the power of 10 is multiplied by the exponent. Therefore, $(3.1 \times 10^2)^2 = 3.1^2 \times 10^{2 \times 2} = 9.6 \times 10^4$.

19. **Q** **What is $(7.25 \times 10^1)^3$?**
    A $7.25^3 = 7.25 \times 7.25 \times 7.25 = 381$
    $10^{1 \times 3} = 10^3$
    $(7.25 \times 10^1)^3 = 3.81 \times 10^5$.

20. **Q** **Divide 6.1×10^2 by 3.4×10^1.**
    A The rule for division with numbers in scientific notation states that the exponent in the denominator is subtracted from the exponent in the numerator. Therefore,
    $$\frac{6.1 \times 10^2}{3.4 \times 10^1} = \frac{6.1 \times 10^{2-1}}{3.4} = 1.8 \times 10^1.$$

21. **Q** **Divide 4.7×10^{-2} by 9.38×10^{-3}.**
    A $\dfrac{4.7 \times 10^{-2}}{9.38 \times 10^{-3}} = \dfrac{4.7 \times 10^{-2-(-3)}}{9.38} = 0.50 \times 10^1 = 5.0$.

22. **Q** **Add 9.3×10^3 to 7.2×10^2.**
    A When adding numbers in scientific notation, first convert the numbers to their nonscientific notation form. In this problem, $9.3 \times 10^3 = 9300$, and $7.2 \times 10^2 = 720$. If you are using a calculator, enter 9.3, press the EXP function key, press 3, and then press ENTER or the equals sign. Then save that number (9300) in the memory of the calculator and enter 7.2×10^2 in the same manner. Perform the addition by recalling 9300 to be added to 720. The sum is 10,020 or 1.0×10^4.

23. **Q** Add 1.1×10^{-2} to 8.9×10^{-1}.

    A $1.1 \times 10^{-2} = 0.011$
    $8.9 \times 10^{-1} = 0.89$
    $0.011 + 0.89 = 0.90$.

24. **Q** Subtract 8.0×10^2 from 7.3×10^3.

    A When subtracting numbers in scientific notation, first convert the numbers to their nonscientific notation. In this problem, $8.0 \times 10^2 = 800$, and $7.3 \times 10^3 = 7300$. If you are using a scientific calculator, enter 8.0, press the EXP function key, press 2, and then press ENTER or the equals sign. Then save that number (800) in the memory of the calculator and enter 7.3×10^3 in the same manner. Perform the subtraction by recalling 800 to be subtracted from 7300. The product is 6500 or 6.5×10^3.

25. **Q** Subtract 4.1×10^{-1} from 3.7×10^{-1}.

    A Convert both terms into their nonscientific notation form. In this problem, $4.1 \times 10^{-1} = 0.41$, and $3.7 \times 10^{-1} = 0.37$.
    $0.37 - 0.41 = -0.04$ or -4.0×10^{-2}.

PRACTICE PROBLEMS

Solve the following problems to further master the material. All answers and explanations to some problems can be found in a separate section at the back of the book.

Determine how many significant figures occur in each of the following numbers.

1. 926.9
2. 707
3. 123.06
4. 0.0402
5. 0.82610
6. 338.00

Solve the following equations. Correct answers must contain the required number of significant figures.

7. $15.6 + 29.4 + 215.83 + 98.1$ = ?
8. $52.5 + 44.99$ = ?
9. $125.957 - 31.22$ = ?
10. $0.032 - 0.005$ = ?

11. 211.5×2.48 $= \ ?$
12. 1.395×2.898 $= \ ?$
13. $3.68 \div 0.94$ $= \ ?$
14. $15.2 \div 3.7$ $= \ ?$

Round the following numbers to three significant figures.
15. 0.6824
16. 12.84
17. 4.162
18. 3.339
19. 5.558
20. 2.635
21. 7.825

Express the following numbers in exponent form.
22. 9365.3
23. 712.0
24. 2000.0
25. 0.2541
26. 0.000822
27. 0.00000477

Solve the following equations using the rules for working with exponents. Answers must be in correct exponent form.
28. $[(9.62 \times 10^3) \, (4.21 \times 10^2)]$
29. $[(3.95 \times 10^4) \, (4.44 \times 10^1)]$
30. $[(6.91 \times 10^{-3}) \, (9.58 \times 10^1)]$
31. $[(4.14 \times 10^{-2}) \, (1.32 \times 10^{-3})]$
32. $[5.5 \times 10^3]^2$
33. $[3.3 \times 10^6]^3$
34. $[7.7 \times 10^{-2}]^2$
35. $[1.7 \times 10^{-3}]^3$
36. $(8.6 \times 10^4) \div (3.1 \times 10^2)$
37. $(2.31 \times 10^2) \div (8.9 \times 10^1)$
38. $(9.235 \times 10^{-3}) \div (1.814 \times 10^{-3})$
39. $(2.6 \times 10^{-4}) \div (6.2 \times 10^{-3})$
40. $(6.66 \times 10^1) + (2.25 \times 10^2)$
41. $(2.7 \times 10^{-2}) + (8.9 \times 10^{-3})$
42. $(4.5 \times 10^3) - (6.3 \times 10^2)$
43. $(3.5 \times 10^{-2}) - (5.7 \times 10^{-3})$

CHAPTER 3

Fractions, Percentages, Ratio, and Proportion

OBJECTIVES

Upon completion of this chapter, the reader should be able to:

1 State the components of a fraction.

2 Perform addition, subtraction, multiplication, and division calculations involving fractions.

3 Convert between simple and compound fractions.

4 Perform addition, subtraction, multiplication, and division calculations involving mixed fractions.

5 Convert fractions into decimal form.

6 Convert numbers between their decimal and percentage forms.

7 Perform ratio and proportion calculations.

INTRODUCTION

Simple Fractions

Fractions are a way of expressing mathematically the relationship between parts of a unit and the unit as a whole. A common illustration of the concept of fractions is a whole pie and its individual slices. The pie itself can be expressed mathematically as a unit of 1. However, the individual slices, which represent only parts of the pie, must be expressed as a unit smaller than 1. Fractions are one way to express this smaller unit. For example, Figure 3-1 illustrates a pie cut in half. How many pieces are there now to the pie?

As you can see, there are two pieces to the pie. The relationship of these two pieces to the whole pie can be expressed mathematically as the fraction ½, or one whole divided into two pieces.

Fractions always consist of two parts. The *numerator* is the top number of the fraction and describes the quantity of the whole unit. In simple fractions, it is the number 1. The *denominator* is the bottom number of the fraction and describes the number of parts comprising the whole unit. In the above example, the denominator is 2.

Therefore, all fractions consist of a numerator and a denominator.

PROBLEMS

In the fraction ¼, what is the numerator and what is the denominator?
The numerator is the top number of the fraction, or 1, and the denominator is the bottom number of the fraction, or 4.

In the fraction ⅓, what is the numerator and what is the denominator?
The numerator is 1, and the denominator is 3. Remember, the numerator is the top number of the fraction, and the denominator is the bottom number.

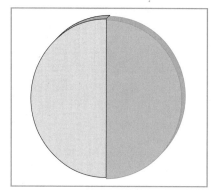

FIGURE 3-1 Pie divided in half.

Simple fractions are fractions such as ⅓, ¼, and ⅛. These fractions all are mathematically as low, or simple, as they can be. No other numbers can be divided into them to make a comparable fraction. Looking at these fractions, picture a pie that is divided into thirds, fourths, or eighths. (see Fig. 3-2)

In general, no matter how complex a mathematic equation may be, it is customary to reduce the final result to its simplest term.

This example also demonstrates that in fractions with the same numerator, the fraction with the lowest denominator is actually the largest fraction. Figures 3-2A to 3-2C show the fractions ⅓, ¼, and ⅛. All have the same numerator, 1, but the fraction ⅓ has the lowest denominator (3) compared to 4 and 8. However, the fraction ⅓ is actually larger than ¼ or ⅛.

Compound Fractions

Compound fractions are fractions in which the numerator and the denominator are divisible by whole numbers. They differ from simple fractions by the fact that the numerator and denominator can be divided by other numbers to reduce these fractions to simple terms. For example, the fraction ²⁄₄ can be reduced to ½ by dividing both the numerator and the denominator by 2, the whole number common to both. In order to reduce a fraction, both the numerator and the denominator must be divided by the same number—in this example, the number 2.

The reduced fraction and the original fraction represent the same proportion of pieces to the whole pie. This is demonstrated in Figures 3-3A and 3-3B, where each piece is represented by the color green.

Each fraction contains the same total area, but it is divided into different numbers of pieces. Figure 3-3A is divided into two pieces, i.e., ½, while Figure 3-3B is divided into four pieces, with two of these pieces shaded green. This is represented as ²⁄₄. However, as you can see, the total area represented by the shaded color in each fraction is the same, showing that ½ and ²⁄₄ are comparable fractions representing the same piece of the pie.

PROBLEMS

Reduce ⁵⁄₂₅ to its simplest form.

The first step when reducing fractions is to find a number that is common to both the numerator and the denominator. In this case, the denominator, 25, is divisible by the numerator, 5. To reduce the fraction, both the numerator and the denominator are divided by the common number, 5, to yield the reduced fraction ⅕. The common number, 5, is called the *common denominator,* or *number common to both parts of the fraction.*

$$\frac{5}{25} \div \frac{5}{5} = \frac{1}{5}$$

Therefore, the fraction ⁵⁄₂₅ is comparable to the fraction ⅕.

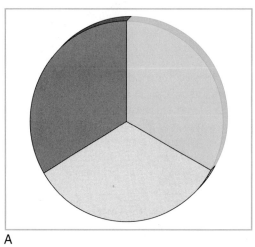

A

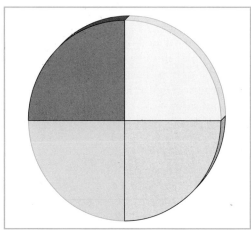

B

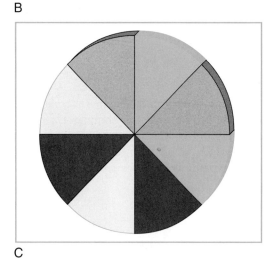

C

FIGURE 3-2 Pie divided in thirds (*A*), fourths (*B*), and eighths (*C*).

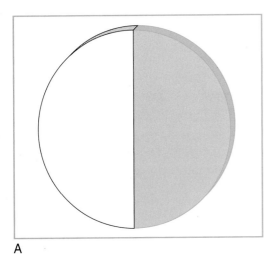　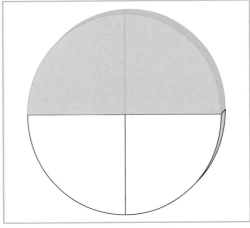

A　　　　　　　　　　　　　　　　　　　　B

FIGURE 3-3　*A*, Two pieces, or ¹/₂; *B*, Four pieces, or ²/₄.

Reduce ²/₈ to its simplest terms.

Remember, the first step is to find the common denominator. One simple method is to determine if the denominator of the fraction is divisible by the numerator. In this instance, 8 is divisible by 2 to yield the common denominator of 4. Therefore, the fraction can be reduced to ¹/₄.

Sometimes fractions involved in equations have different denominators. Before any addition or subtraction calculation is attempted, the fractions must be converted into comparable fractions using the common denominator method.

PROBLEMS

Determine the common denominator for ¹/₃ and ¹/₄.

The simplest method to determine the common denominator is to multiply the denominators of each fraction together to obtain the common denominator:

$3 \times 4 = 12$

The common denominator is 12.

Convert the fractions ¹/₃ and ¹/₄ into comparable fractions.

Since the common denominator has been determined, next multiply the numerator of each fraction by the number used to convert the denominator of each fraction into the common denominator.

To convert the fraction ¼: Since 4 was multiplied by 3 to obtain the common denominator, 12, the numerator for this fraction is multiplied by 3:

$$\frac{1}{12} \times 3 = \frac{3}{12}$$

To convert the fraction ⅓: Since 3 was multiplied by 4 to obtain the common denominator, 12, the numerator for this fraction is multiplied by 4:

$$\frac{1}{12} \times 4 = \frac{4}{12}$$

Therefore, the fractions ⅓ and ¼ are converted into the comparable fractions ⁴/₁₂ and ³/₁₂, respectively.

This example also demonstrates that when two fractions have the same denominator but different numerators, the fraction with the higher numerator is the larger fraction. In this case, ⁴/₁₂ is larger than ³/₁₂.

Adding Fractions

Sometimes two fractions must be added together to determine the sum. As mentioned previously, to be added, the fractions must have the same denominator, i.e., have the same-size pie, or base. If the denominators are not the same, then additional steps must be taken to convert the fractions into comparable units. Figure 3-4 is an example of two fractions with the same denominator added together to determine the sum. The green segment of each fraction is the numerator for that fraction, and the number of pieces in each pie is each fraction's denominator.

Each pie is divided into four pieces; therefore, the first pie can be expressed mathematically as ¼, or one green piece, and the second pie can be expressed mathematically as ²/₄, or two green pieces. The sum is ¾, or three green pieces.

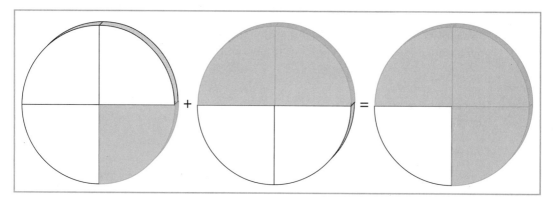

FIGURE 3-4 The sum of ¼ and ²/₄ is ¾.

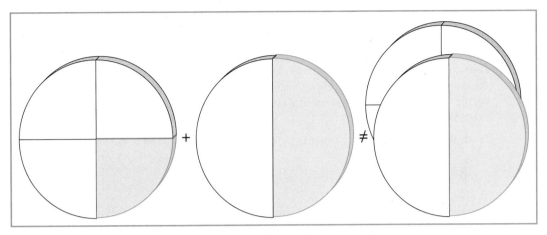

FIGURE 3-5 The fractions ¼ and ½ cannot be added until there is a common denominator.

This example demonstrates why all fractions in the equation must have a common denominator. Note that the second fraction, ²/₄, could have been reduced to its simplest term, ½. Figure 3-5 demonstrates graphically the equation in Figure 3-4, but with the ²/₄ in its simplest terms.

Figure 3-5 shows that because the pieces of the pie in each fraction are different, they cannot be added together.

PROBLEMS

Add ³/₈ and ²/₈.

Because both fractions have the same denominator, to solve this problem simply add the numerators together:

3 + 2 = 5

Therefore, the sum is ⁵/₈.

Add ¼ and ³/₅.

Because the denominators are different, the first step is to determine the common denominator. A simple way is to multiply the denominators of the two fractions:

4 × 5 = 20

Therefore, 20 is the common denominator. Next, each fraction must be converted to its comparable form, with 20 as the denominator. If 20 is the new denominator for each fraction, then each fraction's numerator must be multiplied by the corresponding factor used to convert each fraction's denominator to the number 20.

Let's start with ¼. Since the common denominator has been established as 20, the next step is to convert the numerator. First, look at the relationship between 4 and 20. In order to convert 4 into 20, it must first be multiplied by the factor 5. This same factor must be used to multiply the numerator, 1, to convert it to its comparable form. Therefore, $1 \times 5 = 5$, and the numerator is 5. The comparable fraction is ⁵/₂₀.

Next, convert ³/₅ in the same manner. To convert 5 to the common denominator of 20, the factor 4 is used. Therefore, the numerator, 3, must also be multiplied by the factor 4 to establish the new comparable fraction. Thus $3 \times 4 = 12$, and the new fraction becomes ¹²/₂₀.

Next, since both fractions have a common denominator, the addition can proceed:

$$\frac{5}{20} + \frac{12}{20} = \frac{17}{20}$$

Therefore, the sum of ¼ and ³/₅ is ¹⁷/₂₀.

Add ⅙ and ¼.

To solve this problem, first determine the common denominator. Besides the number 24, the numbers 6 and 4 have the number 12 in common. Therefore, because it is common practice to reduce fractions ultimately to their simplest terms, it is easier to begin the calculations using a lower number. Therefore, 12 will be the common denominator. The next step is to convert each fraction into equivalent terms, as demonstrated in the previous example.

The fraction ⅙ can be converted into ²/₁₂, and the fraction ¼ can be converted into ³/₁₂. Finally, add the two fractions together:

$$\frac{2}{12} + \frac{3}{12} = \frac{5}{12}$$

Therefore, the answer is ⁵/₁₂.

Subtracting Fractions

Calculations involving subtraction of fractions are similar to those involving addition of fractions. All fractions in the calculations must have a common denominator prior to the actual mathematical computation.

PROBLEMS

Subtract ⁹/₁₆ from ¹⁵/₁₆.

Because the denominators of each fraction are the same, i.e., 16, the calculation is straightforward:

$$\frac{15}{16} - \frac{9}{16} = \frac{6}{16}$$

Thus, the answer is ⁶/₁₆, which can be simplified to ³/₈.

Subtract ⅓ from ⅞.

Because the denominators are different, a common denominator may be determined by multiplying the two denominators together to arrive at the common denominator of 24. Next, convert each fraction to its equivalent term by multiplying the numerator of each fraction by the appropriate factor.

$$\frac{1}{3} = \frac{8}{24} \quad \text{and} \quad \frac{7}{8} = \frac{21}{24}$$

Finally, solve the equation:

$$\frac{21}{24} - \frac{8}{24} = \frac{13}{24}$$

Therefore, the answer is ¹³/₂₄.

Subtract ⅕ from ⅘.

Since the denominators of both fractions are the same, i.e., 5, this problem is solved using simple subtraction:

$$\frac{4}{5} - \frac{1}{5} = \frac{3}{5}$$

Therefore, the answer is ³/₅.

Multiplying Fractions

When multiplying fractions, multiply the numerators together and the denominators together. Fractions do not have to have a common denominator, and the calculations can therefore be more straightforward than addition or subtraction calculations.

PROBLEMS

Multiply ⅔ and ¾.

To perform this calculation, multiply both numerators together and both denominators together:

$$\frac{2}{3} \times \frac{3}{4} = \frac{6}{12}$$

The answer, ⁶/₁₂, can be simplified to ½.

Multiply ⁵/₉ and ¾.

Remember, when multiplying fractions, multiply the numerators together and the denominators together to arrive at the answer.

$$\frac{5}{9} \times \frac{3}{4} = \frac{15}{36}$$

The fraction $^{15}/_{36}$ can be reduced by the factor 3 to its simplest terms, $^{5}/_{12}$.

Therefore, the result is $^{5}/_{12}$.

Multiply $^2/_3$ and $^5/_7$.

$$\frac{2}{3} \times \frac{5}{7} = \frac{10}{21}$$

The fraction $^{10}/_{21}$ can be reduced to $^{5}/_{11}$.

Therefore, the result is $^{5}/_{11}$.

Dividing Fractions

Division of fractions is a multistep process. This is because, when dividing fractions, you are actually multiplying. First, state the equation. Then, invert the fraction to the right of the division sign so that the numerator is now the denominator and the denominator is now the numerator. Last, multiply the two fractions together to arrive at the sum.

PROBLEMS

Divide $^1/_5$ by $^1/_3$.

First, set up the division equation:

$$\frac{1}{5} \div \frac{1}{3} = X$$

Next, invert the fraction $^1/_3$ and replace the division sign with a multiplication sign:

$$\frac{1}{5} \times \frac{3}{1} = X$$

Last, using the rules for multiplication of fractions, solve the equation:

$$\frac{1}{5} \times \frac{3}{1} = \frac{3}{5}$$

Therefore, $^1/_5$ divided by $^1/_3$ is $^3/_5$.

Divide $^1/_4$ by $^1/_2$.

Again, first set up the equation:

$$\frac{1}{4} \div \frac{1}{2} = X$$

Then, invert ¼ and multiply by ½ to solve the equation:

$$\frac{1}{4} \times \frac{2}{1} = X$$

$$\frac{2}{4} = X$$

Last, reduce ²⁄₄ to its lowest terms:

$$\frac{2}{4} = \frac{1}{2}$$

Therefore, ¼ divided by ½ is ½.

If you are not sure of your answer to this problem or to any multiplication or division problems involving fractions, double-check your work by performing the opposite calculation on the derived answer. For example, if you're unsure that ¼ divided by ½ is equal to ½, then check your answer by *multiplying* ½ by ½. The result is ¼, which verifies your calculations.

Divide ⁵⁄₁₂ by ³⁄₄.

$$\frac{5}{12} \div \frac{3}{4} = X$$

$$\frac{5}{12} \times \frac{4}{3} = \frac{20}{36}$$

The fraction ²⁰⁄₃₆ can be reduced to its lowest term by dividing it by the factor 4:

$$\frac{20}{36} = \frac{5}{9}$$

Therefore, the answer to this problem is ⁵⁄₉. If you look back at the examples given for multiplication of fractions, you will see that the same fractions were used. This example of a division calculation can be used to check the accuracy of the earlier calculation.

Mixed Fractions

So far, all the examples used in this chapter have involved simple or compound fractions. But what about a fraction such as 1¼ or 1⁵⁄₆? These are mixed fractions, i.e., they contain both a whole number and a fraction. They derive from the simplification of compound fractions in which the numerator is larger than the denominator. Figure 3-6 graphically demonstrates how the fraction ⁵⁄₄ is the same as 1¼.

To convert a mixed fraction into its simplest terms, divide the numerator by the denominator. In the example shown in Figure 3-6, to simplify the fraction ⁵⁄₄, divide the numerator, 5, by the denominator, 4. This results in the fraction 1¼.

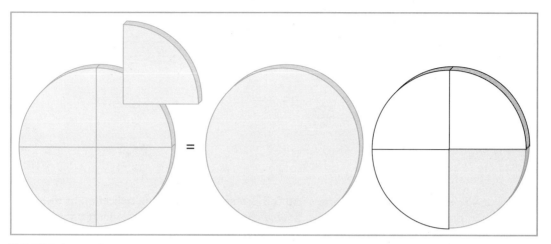

FIGURE 3-6 The fraction ⁵⁄₄ is equal to 1¹⁄₄.

Adding and Subtracting Mixed Fractions

When adding or subtracting mixed fractions, the same rules apply as in addition or subtraction of simple fractions, i.e., the denominators of the fractions must be the same before the calculation can begin. However, the whole numbers associated with each mixed fraction are not changed.

PROBLEMS

Add 1¹⁄₄ and 2⁵⁄₈.

Since the denominators of these fractions are different, the first step is to find the common denominator. In this case, the common denominator is 8, a multiple of the number 4. Next, convert the fraction ¹⁄₄ into its converted form with a denominator of 8: ¹⁄₄ = ²⁄₈.

Next, set up the addition equation:

$$1\frac{2}{8}$$
$$+\ 2\frac{5}{8}$$

Now, add the numerators together:

$$1\frac{2}{8}$$
$$+\ 2\frac{5}{8}$$
$$\frac{7}{8}$$

Last, add the whole numbers together:

$$1\frac{2}{8}$$
$$+\ 2\frac{5}{8}$$
$$\overline{3\frac{7}{8}}$$

Therefore, the sum of 1¼ and 2⅝ is 3⅞.

What is the sum of 3⅗ and 2⅔?

Again, first find the common denominator. The easiest method is to multiply the two denominators together; the result, 15, is the common denominator. Next, convert the numerators to their appropriately converted forms:

$$3\frac{3}{5} = 3\frac{9}{15}$$
$$2\frac{2}{3} = 2\frac{10}{15}$$

Next, add the fractions:

$$3\frac{9}{15}$$
$$+\ 2\frac{10}{15}$$
$$\overline{5\frac{19}{15}}$$

Last, reduce the fraction to its lowest term:

$$5\frac{19}{15} = 6\frac{4}{15}$$

Therefore, the sum of 3⅗ and 2⅔ is 6⁴⁄₁₅.

Solve the following problem: 2⅔ − 1¼.

First, find the common denominator; in this case, it is 12. Then, convert each fraction into its new form:

$$2\frac{2}{3} = 2\frac{8}{12}$$
$$1\frac{1}{4} = 1\frac{3}{12}$$

Next, perform the subtraction:

$$2\frac{8}{12}$$
$$-\,1\frac{3}{12}$$
$$1\frac{5}{12}$$

Thus, 2²/₃ − 1¼ is 1⁵/₁₂.

Subtract 1½ from 2²/₃.

First, find the common denominator for both fractions; in this case, it is 6. Next, convert the fractions into their compound form:

$$1\frac{1}{2} = 1\frac{3}{6}$$
$$2\frac{2}{3} = 2\frac{4}{6}$$

Next, set up and solve the equation:

$$2\frac{4}{6}$$
$$-\,1\frac{3}{6}$$
$$1\frac{1}{6}$$

Therefore, 2¹/₃ − 1½ is 1¹/₆.

Multiplying and Dividing Mixed Fractions

An additional calculation must be performed with mixed fractions before multiplication or division can be done. This calculation converts the mixed fraction into a compound fraction. To convert:

1. Multiply the denominator by the whole number of the fraction.
2. Then add the numerator to form the compound fraction.

PROBLEMS

Convert the mixed fraction 2⅛ into its compound form.

First, multiply the denominator by the whole number:

$$8 \times 2 = 16$$

Next, add the numerator to this number:

$16 + 1 = 17$

Then, place this number as the new numerator:

$$\frac{17}{8}$$

Therefore, $2\frac{1}{8}$ is equal to $\frac{17}{8}$.

Multiply $1\frac{1}{2}$ by $2\frac{2}{3}$.

First, convert each fraction to its compound form:

$$1\frac{1}{2} = \frac{3}{2}$$

$$2\frac{2}{3} = \frac{8}{3}$$

Next, multiply using the rules for multiplication of fractions:

$$\frac{3}{2} \times \frac{8}{3} = \frac{24}{6}$$

Last, reduce $\frac{24}{6}$ to its simplest form. In this case, it becomes the whole number 4.

Multiply $1\frac{7}{8}$ by $2\frac{3}{5}$.

Again, first convert each fraction into its compound form:

$$1\frac{7}{8} = \frac{15}{8}$$

$$2\frac{3}{5} = \frac{13}{5}$$

Now, perform the multiplication calculation:

$$\frac{15}{8} \times \frac{13}{5} = \frac{195}{40}$$

Next, reduce the answer to its simplest form by dividing the numerator and denominator by 5:

$$\frac{195}{40} = \frac{39}{8}$$

Finally, convert the compound fraction into its multiple fraction form:

$$\frac{39}{8} = 4\frac{7}{8}$$

Therefore, $1\frac{7}{8}$ times $2\frac{3}{5}$ is $4\frac{7}{8}$.

Divide 2⅓ by 1¾.

First, convert each fraction into its compound form:

$$2\frac{1}{3} = \frac{7}{3}$$

$$1\frac{3}{4} = \frac{7}{4}$$

Next, perform the division calculation using the rules for division of fractions:

$$\frac{7}{3} \div \frac{7}{4} = X$$

$$\frac{7}{3} \times \frac{4}{7} = X$$

$$\frac{4}{3} = X$$

$$1\frac{1}{3} = X$$

Therefore, 2⅓ divided by 1¾ is 1⅓.

Divide 3³⁄₇ by 2⅔.

First, convert each fraction into its compound form:

$$3\frac{3}{7} = \frac{24}{7}$$

$$2\frac{2}{3} = \frac{8}{3}$$

Next, perform the division calculation:

$$\frac{24}{7} \div \frac{8}{3} = X$$

$$\frac{24}{7} \times \frac{3}{8} = X$$

$$\frac{72}{56} = X$$

$$1\frac{16}{56} = X$$

$$1\frac{2}{7} = X$$

Therefore, 3³⁄₇ divided by 2⅔ is 1²⁄₇.

Converting Fractions into Decimals

In the health care field, a quantity is often expressed in decimal form rather than as a fraction. Like fractions, decimals are based on a total quantity of 1.0, with most decimals being some fraction of 1.0. Converting a fraction to its decimal form is easy; just divide the numerator by the denominator. The final answer will be a number less than 1.0.

PROBLEMS

Convert ½ into its decimal form.

To convert a fraction into its decimal form, divide the numerator by the denominator.

$$2\overline{)1.0}^{\,0.50}$$

Therefore, the fraction ½ is equal to the decimal 0.50.

Convert the fraction ¾ into its decimal form.

To convert, divide the numerator, 3, by the denominator, 4.

$$4\overline{)3.00}^{\,0.75}$$

Therefore, the fraction ¾ is equal to the decimal 0.75.

Convert the fraction ⅔ into its decimal form.

Again, divide the numerator by the denominator:

$$3\overline{)2.00}^{\,0.66}$$

Therefore, the fraction ⅔ is equal to the decimal 0.66.

Converting Decimals into Percentages

Sometimes quantities are listed not as fractions or decimals but as percentages. Percentages are fractions with a constant denominator of 100 and are the ratio of the quantity of a substance per 100 total parts. For example, bleach used for decontamination is at a concentration of 10%; ethanol (EtOH) may be set at a concentration of 75%. The 10% bleach is a ratio of 10 parts bleach per 100 total parts. A 75% EtOH solution may be prepared by placing 75 mL of EtOH in a 100 mL volumetric flask and then adding 25 mL of water for the remaining volume.

It is easy to convert from a decimal into its percentage form. Since a decimal is in the form _.__, simply move the decimal point two places to the right and add a percentage sign. This is a shortcut method of conversion. What you are, in fact, doing is multiplying the decimal by 100.

PROBLEMS

Convert the decimal 0.50 into its percentage form.

The decimal 0.50 can be multiplied by 100 to convert it into its percentage form.

   $0.50 \times 100 = 50\%$

Alternatively, the decimal 0.50 can have its decimal point moved two places to the right to convert it into its percentage form.

   $0.50 = 50\%$

$$0 \,.\, 5\,0 = 50\%$$

Convert 0.24 into its percentage form.

   $0.24 = 24\%$

$$0 \,.\, 2\,4 = 24\%$$

Ratio and Proportion

Health care professionals perform many calculations using the concepts of ratio and proportion. Whenever a different quantity, but *not* a different concentration, of a substance is required, ratio and proportion calculations are performed. A ratio is the relationship of one value to another. A 1:1 ratio represents an equal relationship, while a 1:2 ratio means that one value is twice that of the other. Ratio and proportion is used when a new quantity of a substance is required and is based on an existing ratio. Calculating equivalent fractions is an example of ratio and proportion. For example, the fraction ²/₄ can be converted to its equivalent, ⁴/₈, by the following equation:

Old fraction $\dfrac{2}{4} = \dfrac{X}{8}$ New fraction

By cross-multiplying the numerator of ²/₄ with the denominator of ˣ/₈ and the denominator of ²/₄ with the numerator of ˣ/₈, the equation can be solved:

   $(2)(8) = (X)(4)$
   $16 = (4)(X)$

When both sides of the equation are divided by $\frac{1}{4}$, the equation becomes:

$$\frac{16}{4} = X$$

$$4 = X$$

Thus, $\frac{2}{4}$ is equivalent to $\frac{4}{8}$ because the basic concentration of both fractions is the same.

PROBLEMS

 A medical assistant in a busy internal medicine practice was instructed to give a patient a 250 mg dose of ibuprofen. The drug came from the manufacturer in tablet form in a dose of 500 mg per tablet. How should the medical assistant dispense this dose?

To solve this problem, use ratio and proportion.

First, the medical assistant determines what information is available. The drug is available in a dose of 500 mg per tablet. This can be expressed mathematically as:

$$\frac{500 \text{ mg}}{1 \text{ tablet}}$$

Next, she determines what she wants. The medical assistant wants to know how many tablets to give this patient to dispense a 250 mg dose.

Therefore, if $\dfrac{500 \text{ mg}}{1 \text{ tablet}}$ then $\dfrac{250 \text{ mg}}{X \text{ tablet}}$

Use ratio and proportion to solve this problem. This is accomplished by cross-multiplying this equation to yield the following:

$$\frac{500 \text{ mg}}{1 \text{ tablet}} = \frac{250 \text{ mg}}{X \text{ tablet}}$$

$$(500)(X) = (250)(1)$$

$$X = \frac{250}{500}$$

$$X = \frac{1}{2}$$

Therefore, to give a 250 mg dose using a tablet that contains 500 mg per tablet, the medical assistant gives the patient one-half of one tablet.

Many students find it easier to use the following formula:

$$\frac{\text{What you want}}{\text{What you have}} \times \underset{\text{(DF)}}{\text{Drug form}} = \underset{\text{(ADD)}}{\text{Amount of dispensed drug}}$$

This calculation is easiest to use when the DF is a tablet, capsule, and so on. Some students find it confusing to use this formula when the method of delivery is in a solution with a quantity such as X amount mg/mL.

A nurse practitioner wanted to administer 500 mg of Aldomet to a patient. The drug is available in 250 mg tablets. How should the nurse practitioner administer the correct drug dosage?

Use the above formula to solve this problem by remembering the following:

$$\frac{\text{What you want}}{\text{What you have}} \times \underset{\text{(DF)}}{\text{Drug form}} = \underset{\text{(ADD)}}{\text{Amount of dispensed drug}}$$

The equation to solve this problem becomes:

$$\frac{1000 \text{ mg of drug (what you want)}}{500 \text{ mg of drug per tablet (what you have)}} \times 1 \text{ tablet} = \text{Amt. of dispensed drug}$$

Solving the equation:

two tablets = amount of dispensed drug

Therefore, the nurse practitioner would give the patient two tablets of the drug to administer the ordered dose of 500 mg.

Additional ratio and proportion drug calculations are found in Chapters 7 and 8.

EXAMPLE PROBLEMS

This section is designed to be useful to both the student and the health care practitioner. Students can use the example problems in order to master the material. The health care practitioner can use these problems as templates for solving calculations. Find an example problem similar to the problem that you need to solve and substitute into the equation the numbers appropriate to your calculation.

1. **Q** **What is the name of the top number of a fraction?**
   A The top number of a fraction is called the numerator.

2. **Q** **What is the name of the bottom number of a fraction?**
   A The bottom number of a fraction is called the denominator.

3. **Q** **Given the fraction ³⁄₈, what is the value of the numerator and what is the value of the denominator?**
   A The value of the numerator is 3, and the value of the denominator is 8.

4. **Q** **Reduce the fraction ⁶⁄₈ to its simplest terms.**
   A Reducing a fraction means converting it into a fraction whose numbers are not divisible by any other whole number. To reduce a frac-

tion, first determine what number is common to both the numerator and the denominator. This shared number is called the common denominator. In this case, 2 is the common denominator. Next, divide both the numerator and the denominator by the common denominator, 2, to yield the reduced fraction $3/8$.

5. Q **Reduce the fraction $15/25$ to its simplest terms.**

A The fraction can be reduced to $3/5$.

6. Q **Determine the common denominator for the fractions $1/6$ and $1/5$.**

A The simplest way to determine a common denominator is to multiply both denominators together. Therefore, the common denominator is 30.

7. Q **Add the fractions $1/7$ and $3/7$.**

A To add fractions with similar denominators, simply add the numerators:

$$1/7 + 3/7 = 4/7.$$

8. Q **Add the fractions $1/6$ and $1/5$.**

A Fractions must have a common or similar denominator before addition calculations can be performed. Example question 6 showed how a common denominator is found using these fractions. The common denominator was determined to be 30. After the common denominator has been determined, the numerator of each fraction must be converted to its equivalent value. Starting with the fraction $1/6$, since the denominator will be converted to 30, the numerator must be multiplied by 5, which was used to convert the denominator, 6, to the common denominator, 30. Therefore, the fraction $5/30$ is equal to the original fraction, $1/6$. Next, the fraction $1/5$ is converted to its equivalent term. Since the denominator, 5, was multiplied by 6 to become the common denominator, 30, the numerator must also be multiplied by 5. Therefore, $1/5$ becomes $5/30$. Now that both fractions have a common denominator, the addition calculation can be performed:

$$5/30 + 6/30 = 11/30.$$

Therefore, $1/6 + 1/5 = 11/30$.

9. Q **Add the fractions $2/3$ and $1/2$.**

A The common denominator for these fractions is 6. Therefore, to convert $2/3$ to its comparable fraction with a denominator of 6, the numerator and the denominator must be multiplied by the factor of 2. This factor is used because 3 goes into 6 two times. Therefore, $2/3$ is equal to $4/6$. To convert the fraction $1/2$, both the numerator and the denominator are multiplied by a factor of 3 to yield the equivalent fraction of $3/6$. Last, the equivalent fractions are added:

$4/6 + 3/6 = 7/6.$

$7/6$ can be reduced to $1 1/6$.

10. **Q** **Add the fractions $3/4$ and $2/5$.**

A The sum of $3/4$ and $2/5$ is determined by the following equation:

$15/20 + 8/20 = 23/20$ or $1 3/20$.

11. **Q** **Subtract $4/7$ from $6/7$.**

A As with addition of fractions, since the denominators are common, the numerator 4 is subtracted from the numerator 6 to yield a product of $2/7$.

12. **Q** **Subtract $3/8$ from $2/3$.**

A As with addition of fractions, the denominators must be the same number before subtraction can be performed. Therefore, the fractions must be converted to equivalent fractions first. Since the common denominator is 24, $3/8$ becomes $9/24$ and $2/3$ becomes $16/24$. The subtraction calculation is:

$16/24 - 9/24 = 7/24$.

13. **Q** **Subtract $4/5$ from $7/8$.**

A The equivalent equation for this problem is:

$35/40 - 32/40 = 3/40$.

14. **Q** **Multiply the fractions $4/5$ and $7/8$.**

A When multiplying fractions, the numerators are multiplied together and the denominators are multiplied together. Therefore, the equation is:

$4/5 \times 7/8 = 28/40 = 7/10$.

15. **Q** **Multiply the fractions $2/3$ and $9/16$.**

A $2/3 \times 9/16 = 18/48 = 3/8$.

16. **Q** **Divide $2/3$ by $1/4$.**

A To perform a division calculation, first state the equation:

$2/3 \div 1/4$

Next, invert the fraction to the right of the division sign so that the numerator is now the denominator:

$2/3 \div 4/1$

Last, change the division sign to a multiplication sign and multiply the two fractions together to arrive at the sum.

$2/3 \times 1/4 = 2/12 = 1/6$.

17. **Q** **Divide $5/6$ by $2/3$.**

    A This calculation is solved by the following equation:

    $5/6 \times 3/2 = 15/12 = 1 1/4$.

18. **Q** **Add $2 2/5$ and $1 1/4$.**

    A Fractions consisting of a mixture of a whole number and a fraction are called mixed fractions. When solving addition or subtraction problems that contain mixed fractions, the same basic rule applies, i.e., the denominator must be the same for all fractions in the problem. However, the whole numbers associated with the mixed fraction are not changed before the calculation begins. Therefore, this equation is solved as follows:

    $2 2/5 + 1 1/4 = X$.

    Since a common denominator must be found, these fractions are converted into the following forms:

    $2 8/20 + 1 5/20 = X$.

    Add only the numerators: $8/20 + 5/20 = 13/20$.

    Add the whole numbers: $2 + 1 = 3$.

    Combine the whole number with the fraction to arrive at the sum:

    $3 13/20$.

19. **Q** **Add $1 1/4$ and $3 5/8$.**

    A $1 2/8 + 3 5/8 = 4 7/8$.

20. **Q** **Subtract $1 3/4$ from $2 4/5$.**

    A This problem is solved by the following equation:

    $2 4/5 - 1 3/4 = X$.

    $2 16/20 - 1 15/20 = X$.

    $1 1/20 = X$.

21. **Q** **Subtract $2 2/3$ from $3 3/8$.**

    A $3 9/24 - 2 16/24 = X$.

    The number $3 9/24$ is larger than $2 16/24$ even though 9 is not larger than 16. Instead of subtracting 16 from 9, reduce the whole number 3 by a factor of 1, or $24/24$, "borrowing" this $24/24$ to add to the $9/24$. Therefore, $3 9/24$ is equal to $2 33/24$.

    $2 33/24 - 2 16/24 = 17/24$.

22. **Q** **Multiply $2 3/5$ by $4 5/8$.**

    A In order to multiply or divide mixed fractions, first convert them into compound fractions. This is accomplished by a two-step process. First, multiply the denominator by the whole number to arrive at a product. Next, add the original numerator to the product to arrive at the numerator for the new compound fraction.

$2^3/_5 = 2 \times 5 = 10 + 3 = {}^{13}/_5.$
$4^5/_8 = 4 \times 8 = 32 + 5 = {}^{37}/_8.$
${}^{13}/_5 \times {}^{37}/_8 = X.$
${}^{481}/_{40} = X.$
${}^{481}/_{40}$ is reduced to $12^1/_{40}.$
Therefore, $2^3/_5$ times $4^5/_8$ is $12^1/_{40}.$

23. **Q Multiply $1^1/_3$ by $2^4/_5.$**

   A $1^1/_3 \times 2^4/_5 = X.$
   $^4/_3 \times {}^{14}/_5 = X.$
   ${}^{56}/_{15} = X.$
   $3^{11}/_{15} = X.$

24. **Q Divide $2^1/_3$ by $1^1/_4.$**

   A The mixed fractions in a division calculation are converted to their compound form before division is performed:
   $2^1/_3 \div 1^1/_4 = X.$
   $^7/_3 \div {}^5/_4 = X.$
   $^7/_3 \times {}^4/_5 = X.$
   ${}^{28}/_{15} = X.$
   $1^{13}/_{15} = X.$

25. **Q Divide $3^3/_4$ by $1^1/_2.$**

   A Convert the mixed fractions to their compound form before performing any other calculation:
   $3^3/_4 \div 1^1/_2 = X.$
   ${}^{15}/_4 \div {}^3/_2 = X.$
   Next, perform the division calculation:
   ${}^{15}/_4 \times {}^2/_3 = X.$
   ${}^{30}/_{12} = X.$
   Last, reduce the fraction ${}^{30}/_{12}$ to its lowest terms:
   ${}^{30}/_{12} = 2^1/_2.$

26. **Q Convert $^3/_4$ to its decimal form.**

   A To convert a fraction to its decimal form, divide the numerator by the denominator:
   $3 \div 4 = 0.75.$
   Therefore, $^3/_4$ is equal to 0.75.

27. **Q Convert $^5/_6$ to its decimal form.**

   A $5 \div 6 = 0.83.$
   Therefore, $^5/_6$ is equal to 0.83.

28. **Q** **Convert the decimal 0.66 to its percentage form.**

    A To convert a decimal to its percentage form, multiply the decimal by 100:

      $0.66 \times 100 = 66\%$.

29. **Q** **Convert the decimal 0.75 to its percentage form.**

    A $0.75 \times 100 = 75\%$.

30. **Q** **An order was written for a patient to receive 30 mg/kg/day of amoxicillin. The patient weighed 55 kg. How much drug should the patient receive daily?**

    A Ratio and proportion can be used to solve this problem. The order of 30 mg/kg means that for every kilogram of body weight, the patient receives 30 mg of the drug. Therefore, the following formula can be used:

$$\frac{30 \text{ mg}}{1 \text{ kg}} = \frac{X \text{ mg}}{55 \text{ kg}}$$

Solving the equation:

      $X = (30)(55)$

         $= 1650$ mg or 1.65 g.

31. **Q** **If a dose of 0.75 g of amoxicillin is ordered and the drug comes in the form of scored tablets containing 500 mg of the drug, how many tablets should the patient be given?**

    A This problem can be solved using ratio and proportion. Ratio and proportion calculations can be used when the quantity, but not the concentration, of a substance, i.e., the drug or solution, needs to be changed. An easy way to remember what to do is to recall the following formula:

$$\frac{\text{What you want}}{\text{What you have}} \times \underset{\text{(DF)}}{\text{Drug form}} = \underset{\text{(ADD)}}{\text{Amount of dispensed drug}}$$

Since 0.75 g of the drug is what we want, and what we have is the drug in 500 mg tablets, first convert the number of grams of amoxicillin that are ordered into milligrams:

      0.75 g $= 750$ mg.

Next, substitute the known values into the equation:

$$\frac{750 \text{ (Want)}}{500 \text{ (Have)}} \times 1 \text{ tablet} = \text{ADD}$$

      $1.5 = \text{ADD}$.

Therefore, the patient would be given $1\frac{1}{2}$ 500 mg tablets to meet the drug dosage requirement.

PRACTICE PROBLEMS

Solve the following practice problems to further master the material. All answers and explanations to some problems can be found in a separate section at the back of the book.

For each of the following fractions, determine which number is the numerator and which number is the denominator.

1. $\frac{1}{2}$
2. $\frac{5}{6}$
3. $\frac{4}{6}$
4. $\frac{1}{3}$

Reduce the following fractions to their simplest forms.

5. $\frac{5}{25}$
6. $\frac{4}{8}$
7. $\frac{2}{6}$
8. $\frac{6}{30}$
9. Determine the common denominator for the fractions $\frac{3}{4}$ and $\frac{2}{3}$.
10. Determine the common denominator for the fractions $\frac{5}{6}$ and $\frac{1}{2}$.

Solve the following equations.

11. $\frac{1}{2} + \frac{3}{4}$
12. $\frac{1}{8} + \frac{5}{8}$
13. $\frac{4}{5} + \frac{1}{2}$
14. $\frac{2}{5} + \frac{1}{3}$
15. $\frac{4}{5} - \frac{2}{5}$
16. $\frac{3}{4} - \frac{1}{3}$
17. $\frac{7}{8} - \frac{1}{4}$
18. $\frac{1}{2} - \frac{1}{4}$
19. $\frac{1}{3} \times \frac{2}{5}$
20. $\frac{4}{5} \times \frac{7}{8}$
21. $\frac{1}{2} \times \frac{1}{2}$
22. $\frac{2}{3} \times \frac{1}{2}$
23. $\frac{1}{3} \div \frac{1}{4}$
24. $\frac{9}{15} \div \frac{1}{2}$
25. $1\frac{2}{3} + 2\frac{3}{8}$
26. $2\frac{1}{4} + 3\frac{5}{6}$
27. $2\frac{1}{3} - 1\frac{1}{5}$
28. $1\frac{7}{8} - 1\frac{1}{3}$
29. $2\frac{4}{5} \times 1\frac{5}{6}$

30. $1^{1}/_{4} \times 2^{2}/_{3}$
31. $3^{4}/_{5} \div 2^{2}/_{5}$
32. $2^{1}/_{3} \div 1^{1}/_{4}$

Convert the following fractions into decimal form.
33. $^{2}/_{3}$
34. $^{5}/_{6}$
35. $^{1}/_{2}$

Convert the following decimals into percent form.
36. 0.75
37. 0.22
38. 0.10
39. A nurse practitioner wrote a prescription for a 0.50 mg dose of a drug. When she went to the medication cabinet to obtain the drug, she found that it was available only in 0.25 mg tablets. How did the nurse practitioner dispense the drug?
40. A pharmacist received an order for a certain drug to be given to a patient in a dose of 250 mg. The only available form of the drug is scored 500 mg tablets. How did the pharmacist dispense the drug?

CHAPTER 4

Systems of Measurement

INTRODUCTION

Measurement of Length, Weight, and Mass

U.S. Customary System

Systems of weights and measures have been in existence since the first trade occurred among prehistoric peoples. The Egyptians used the cubit, which may be the earliest known use of linear measurement. One cubit was the distance between the elbow and the tip of the little finger. Later, the Greeks and Romans adopted many of the measurements used in the Egyptian system. The U.S. Customary System of measurement is based on the English system, which draws largely from the Greek and Roman systems. The United States is one of a handful of countries that still use this system. Scientists and most other countries prefer the metric system. However, in the United States, efforts to persuade the public to adopt the metric system have not succeeded. Americans want their foot-long hot dogs, their gallons of milk, and their miles of road. However, change may come from the business community as international trade agreements mandate the use of the metric system as the standard for measurements.

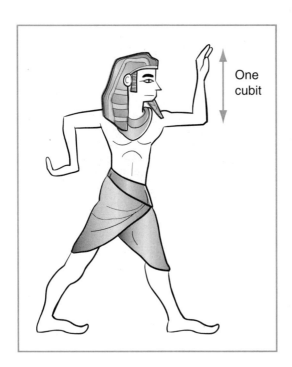

One cubit

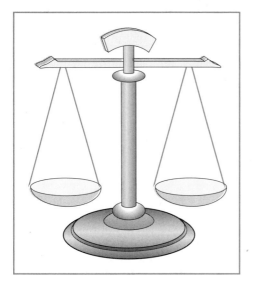

U.S. Customary System of Measurement of Length and Area

Measurement of length in the U.S. Customary System begins with the inch and progresses to the mile and acre.

12 inches	=	1 foot
3 feet (36 inches)	=	1 yard
220 yards	=	1 furlong
8 furlongs	=	1 mile
1760 yards	=	1 mile
5280 feet	=	1 mile
1 square foot	=	144 square inches
1 square yard	=	9 square feet
43,560 square feet	=	1 acre
1 square mile	=	640 acres

U.S. Customary System of Liquid or Dry Measurement

Measurement of liquids begins with the teaspoon and progresses to the gallon.

1 teaspoon	=	1/3 tablespoon	5$\frac{1}{3}$ fluid ounces	=	2/3 cup
2 tablespoons	=	1 fluid ounce	6 fluid ounces	=	3/4 cup
1 fluid ounce	=	1/8 cup	8 fluid ounces	=	1 cup
2 fluid ounces	=	1/4 cup	2 cups	=	1 pint
2$\frac{2}{3}$ fluid ounces	=	1/3 cup	2 liquid pints	=	1 liquid quart
4 fluid ounces	=	1/2 cup	4 liquid quarts	=	1 gallon

Measurements of dry volumes include the following.

1 dry quart	=	2 dry pints
8 dry pints	=	1 peck
4 pecks	=	1 bushel

U.S. Customary System for Measurement of Mass

Currently, four different measurement systems are used in the United States to measure weight:

Troy: used to weigh silver, gold, and other precious metals
Apothecaries: used by pharmacists to weigh drugs
Avoirdupois: used for general purposes
Metric system: used in science and medicine

TROY

1 pennyweight	=	24 grains
20 pennyweights	=	1 ounce
12 ounces	=	1 pound
5760 grains	=	1 pound
3.2 grains	=	1 carat

APOTHECARIES

1 scruple	=	20 grains
3 scruples	=	1 dram
8 drams	=	1 ounce
12 ounces	=	1 pound
5760 grains	=	1 pound

AVOIRDUPOIS

1 dram	=	$27^{11}/_{32}$ grains
16 drams	=	1 ounce
16 ounces	=	1 pound
7000 grains	=	1 pound
100 pounds	=	1 hundredweight
2000 pounds	=	1 short ton
2240 pounds	=	1 long ton

As you can see, these measurements are not consistent with one another, leading to confusion. It was because of this inconsistency that another method of measurement that could be standardized was sought. That system is the metric system, which was developed in France in the 1790s.

Metric System

The metric system is based on fixed standards and a uniform scale of 10. There are three basic units of measurement for length, weight, and volume:

length	=	meter
mass	=	kilogram
volume	=	liter

The meter (m) is defined as the length of the path traveled by light in a vacuum in $1/299,792,458$ of a second. The kilogram (kg) is defined as the mass of water contained by a cube whose sides are $1/10$ the length of 1 m or 1 decimeter in length. The liter (L) is defined as the volume of liquid contained within that same cube.

Another measurement is area, which is derived from the measurement of length. By multiplying the length by the width of a square surface, the area of the surface can be determined. Area is measured in squared units. Common metric area measurements are the square millimeter (mm^2), square centimeter (cm^2), and square meter (m^2).

Prefixes before the basic units of measurement indicate whether a measurement is larger or smaller than the basic unit. Memorizing the following table of prefixes and their abbreviations shown in Table 4-1 will be helpful in learning the metric system.

TABLE 4-1 Metric System Prefixes and Abbreviations

Prefix	Abbreviation	Comparison to Basic Unit
femto	f	10^{-15} smaller
pico	p	10^{-12} smaller
nano	n	10^{-9} smaller
micro	μ or mc	10^{-6} smaller
milli	m	10^{-3} smaller
centi	c	10^{-2} smaller
deci	d	10^{-1} smaller
deca	da	10^{+1} larger
hecto	h	10^{+2} larger
kilo	k	10^{+3} larger
mega	M	10^{+6} larger

Conversion between Different Measurements within the Metric System

Because the metric system is based on a scale of 10, conversion between different measurements within a unit is relatively simple. A simple ratio and proportion calculation is all that is needed to perform the conversion. Table 4-2 contains common metric units, their abbreviations, and their comparable units.

> **Note** The metric term *micro* (0.000001 or 10^{-6}) tends to be abbreviated as "mc" in the general health care field but as the Greek letter μ in the clinical laboratory. For example, *microgram* is frequently abbreviated as "mcg" for drug dosages but as "μg" in the clinical laboratory.

Most drugs are given in terms of milligrams per milliliter (mg/mL) or micrograms per milliliter (mcg/mL or μg/mL) or by body weight in terms of milligrams per kilogram (mg/kg). In the clinical laboratory, many analytes are measured in terms of milligrams per deciliter (mg/dL), or the number of milligrams contained in 1 dL of whole blood. The concentration of most analytes is usually small; some hormones are measured in terms of nanograms per deciliter (ng/dL) or picograms per deciliter (pg/dL). In hematology, white blood cells were previously

TABLE 4-2 Conversion between Different Metric System Units of Measurement

Unit	Abbreviation		Comparable Unit
1 megameter	Mm	=	1,000,000 or 10^6 meters
1 kilometer	km	=	1000 meters
1 deciliter	dL	=	0.1 or 10^{-1} liters
10 deciliters	dL	=	1 liter
1 centimeter	cm	=	0.01 or 10^{-2} meters
10 centimeters	cm	=	1 decimeter
1 millimeter	mm	=	0.001 or 10^{-3} meters
10 millimeters	mm	=	1 centimeter
1 microgram	μg or mcg	=	0.000001 or 10^{-6} grams
1000 micrograms	μg or mcg	=	1 milligram
1 nanometer	nm	=	0.000000001 or 10^{-9} meters
1000 nanometers	nm	=	1 micrometer
1 picogram	pg	=	0.000000000001 or 10^{-12} grams
1000 picograms	pg	=	1 nanogram
1 femtoliter	fL	=	0.000000000000001 or 10^{-15} liters
1000 femtoliters	fL	=	1 nanoliter
1 square centimeter	cm^2	=	100 mm^2
1 square meter	m^2	=	10,000 mm^2

counted in terms of cubic millimeters (mm³) but are currently expressed in liters. In immunohematology, a unit of blood typically holds approximately ½ L of whole blood.

PROBLEMS

How many milliliters are in a 2 L soda bottle?

In order to convert liters to milliliters, the basic value of each must be known. From the previous chart, 1 mL is 1000 times or 10^{-3} times smaller than the base value of 1 L.

Using ratio and proportion:

$$\frac{1\ L}{1000\ mL} = \frac{2\ L}{X\ L}$$

Cross-multiplying the equation:

$$(1)(X) = (2)(1000)$$
$$X = 2000$$

There are 2000 mL (2×10^3 mL) in a 2 L soda bottle.

How many micrograms are in 3.5 pg?

One microgram is 1×10^{-6} of a gram (g) or 0.000001 g. One picogram is 1000 times smaller than a microgram or 1×10^{-9} g. One picogram can also be expressed as 0.000000001 g. By using ratio and proportion, the units can be converted from one system to the other.

$$\frac{1\ \mu g}{1000\ pg} = \frac{X\ \mu g}{3.5\ pg}$$

Cross-multiplying the equation:

$$(1)(3.5) = (1000)(X)$$
$$3.5 = (1000)(X)$$
$$\frac{3.5}{1000} = X$$
$$0.0035 = X$$
$$3.5 \times 10^{-3} = X$$

Therefore, there are 3.5×10^{-3} μg (mcg) in 3.5 pg.

How many micrograms are in 25 mg?

A microgram is 1×10^{-6} g or 0.000001 g. One milligram is 1000 times larger than 1 μg or 1×10^{-3} g. One milligram can also be expressed as 0.001 g. By using ratio and proportion, the units can be converted from one system to the other.

$$\frac{1 \text{ mg}}{1000 \text{ µg}} = \frac{25 \text{ mg}}{X \text{ µg}}$$

Cross-multiplying the equation:

$$(1)(X) = (1000)(25)$$
$$X = 25000$$

Therefore, there are 25,000 or 2.5×10^4 µg (mcg) in 25 mg.

How many micrograms are in 0.500 mg?

Remember, a microgram is 1×10^{-6} g or 0.000001 g. A milligram is 1000 times larger than a microgram or 1×10^{-3} g. One milligram can also be expressed as 0.001 g. By using ratio and proportion, the units can be converted from one to the other.

$$\frac{1 \text{ mg}}{1000 \text{ µg}} = \frac{0.500 \text{ mg}}{X \text{ µg}}$$

Cross-multiplying the equation:

$$(1)(X) = (1000)(0.500)$$
$$X = 500$$

Therefore, there are 500 µg (mcg) in 0.500 mg.

Shortcut Method for Conversion between Metric System Units

As shown in the example above, because 1 µg is 1000 times smaller than 1 mg, a shortcut method of conversion is to move the decimal point three spaces to the right to convert milligrams to micrograms. For example, moving the decimal point of 0.500 mg three spaces to the right converts it to 500 µg (mcg).

0 . 5 0 0 milligrams = 0 . 5 0 0 = 500 micrograms

Remember that there are 0.0035 µg (mcg) in 3.5 pg. A shortcut method is to move the decimal point of 3.5 pg three spaces to the left to convert it to 0.0035 µg (mcg).

3 . 5 picograms = 0 0 0 3 . 5 = 0.0035 micrograms

Summary. When converting from a larger metric unit to a smaller metric unit, move the decimal point the appropriate number of spaces to the *right*. When converting a smaller metric unit to a larger metric unit, move the decimal point the appropriate number of spaces to the *left*.

PROBLEMS

Using the shortcut method, how many grams are in a 250 mg dose of aspirin?

Because a gram is larger than a milligram, the decimal point is moved three spaces to the left. Therefore, 250 mg of aspirin is equal to 0.250 g of aspirin.

A physician wrote an order for 0.10 g of penicillin. How many milligrams of penicillin are there in 0.10 g?

Using the shortcut method, since the milligram is smaller than a gram, the decimal point is moved three spaces to the left. Therefore, 0.10 g is equal to 100 mg of penicillin.

Conversion between Units within the Metric System

Sometimes a measurement may have to be converted to a different but comparable value in order to perform a calculation. Units can be converted from one form to another if the correct unit conversion fraction is used in the calculation. For example, there are 10 dL in 1 L. Frequently, laboratory results are reported in terms of a deciliter quantity (e.g., mg/dL, g/dL), while drug levels are frequently reported in mg/mL terms. Because there are 10 dL per liter, the quantity in milligrams per liter can be multiplied by 10 to be equivalent to the quantity in liters.

PROBLEMS

Convert 90 mg/dL to the mg/L equivalent.

The value 90 mg/dL can be written as $\dfrac{90 \text{ mg}}{1 \text{ dL}}$.

There are 10 dL in 1 L. Therefore, the fraction 10 dL/1 L = 1.

The rules of algebra allow any number to be multiplied by 1 in an equation. Therefore:

$$\frac{90 \text{ mg}}{1 \text{ dL}} \times \frac{10 \text{ dL}}{1 \text{ L}} = \frac{(90 \text{ mg})(10 \text{ dL})}{(1 \text{ dL})(1 \text{ L})}$$

Cancel the units in the equation:

$$\frac{(90 \text{ mg})(10 \cancel{\text{ dL}})}{(1 \cancel{\text{ dL}})(1 \text{ L})} = \frac{900 \text{ mg}}{1 \text{ L}}$$

The result is 900 mg/L.

TABLE 4-3 Conversion from the U.S. Customary System to the Metric System

Convert from U.S. System (Unit of 1)	Convert to Metric System (Unit of 1)	Multiply by Conversion Factor
inch (in)	millimeter (mm)	25.4
inch (in)	centimeter (cm)	2.54
inch (in)	meter (m)	0.0254
yard (yd)	meter (m)	0.91
mile (mi)	kilometer (km)	1.61
ounce (oz)	gram (g)	28.3
ounce (oz)	milliliter (mL)	29.6
pound (lb)	kilogram (kg)	0.453
pint (pt)	liter (L)	0.474
gallon (gal)	liter (L)	3.79

Convert 1500 µg/mL to the mg/mL equivalent.

Remember, there are 1000 µg (mcg) in 1 mg. Therefore, the fraction 1 mg/1000 µg = 1.

Since a fraction that is equal to 1 can be used on both sides of an equation, the following conversion equation can be determined:

$$\frac{1500\ \mu g}{1\ mL} \times \frac{1\ mg}{1000\ \mu g} = \frac{(1500\ \mu g)(1\ mg)}{(1\ mL)(1000\ \mu g)}$$

Cancel the units in the equation:

$$\frac{(1500\ \cancel{\mu g})(1\ mg)}{(1\ mL)(1000\ \cancel{\mu g})} = 1.5\ mg/mL$$

The result is 1.5 mg/mL.

Conversion between the U.S. Customary System and the Metric System

Since the Customary System is so widely used in the United States, it may be necessary to convert between this system and the metric system. The measurements that are commonly used are listed in Table 4-3.

PROBLEMS

How many milliliters are there in a 16 ounce (oz) soft drink?

From Table 4-3, 1 oz = 29.6 mL. Using ratio and proportion, the following equation is derived:

$$\frac{1\ oz}{29.6\ mL} = \frac{16\ oz}{X\ mL}$$

Cross-multiplying the equation:

$$(1)(X) = (16)(29.6)$$
$$X = 474 \text{ mL}$$

There are 474 mL in a 16 oz soft drink.

Another way to calculate this equation is to multiply 16 oz by the conversion factor of 29.6 to yield 474 mL.

How many milliliters are in 1 tablespoon of cough syrup?

This conversion is a two-step process. First, convert tablespoons to ounces. Then, convert ounces to milliliters. Earlier in this chapter, it was shown that 2 tablespoons equals 1 fluid ounce. Therefore, 1 tablespoon equals 0.5 ounce. Using Table 4-3, the conversion factor is 29.6. Therefore, multiply the number of ounces, 0.5, by 29.6:

$$0.5 \times 29.6 = X$$
$$14.8 = X$$

Therefore, there are 14.8 mL in 1 tablespoon of cough syrup.

How many milliliters are there in 1 teaspoon of pediatric decongestant?

This is also a multistep process. First, convert teaspoons to tablespoons. There are 3 teaspoons in 1 tablespoon. Therefore, a 1 teaspoon dose is a 0.33 tablespoon dose. Next, convert tablespoons to ounces. Remember, 2 tablespoons equals 1 ounce. Using ratio and proportion:

$$\frac{2 \text{ tablespoons}}{1 \text{ oz}} = \frac{0.33 \text{ tablespoons}}{X \text{ oz}}$$
$$(2)(X) = (1)(0.33)$$
$$X = \frac{0.33}{2}$$
$$X = 0.165$$

Therefore, there is 0.165 ounce in 1 teaspoon of cough syrup. Next, use the conversion factor of 29.6 to convert from ounces to milliliters:

$$0.165 \times 29.6 = 4.9 \text{ mL}$$

Therefore, 1 teaspoon of cough syrup is equal to a 4.9 mL dose.

How many pounds are equal to 70 kg?

From Table 4-3, 1 kg is equal to 2.2 lb. Therefore, multiply the number of kilograms by the conversion factor of 2.2:

$$70 \times 2.2 = 154$$

Therefore, 154 lb is equal to 70 kg.

How many kilograms are equal to 225 lb?

From Table 4-3, 1 lb is equal to 0.453 kg. Therefore, multiply the number of pounds by the conversion factor of 0.453 kg.

225 × 0.453 = 102

Therefore, 102 kg is equal to 225 lb.

If a patient is 66 in. tall, what is his height in meters?

Using Table 4-3, 1 in. is equal to 0.0254 m. Therefore, multiply the number of inches by the conversion factor of 0.0254 m.

66 × 0.0254 = 1.7 m

Therefore a patient who is 66 in. tall is 1.7 m tall.

Conversion between the Metric System and the U.S. Customary System

Sometimes a metric unit is converted to a U.S. Customary System measurement. To convert from the metric unit to the U.S. system unit, multiply the metric unit by the conversion factor given in Table 4-4. Note that these conversion factors are the reciprocal of the conversion unit used to convert from the U.S. system to the metric system.

PROBLEMS

If a patient is 2 m tall, what is her height in inches?

From Table 4-4, 1 m is equal to 39.6 in. Multiply the number of meters by the conversion factor of 39.6.

2 m × 39.6 = 79.2 in

Therefore, a patient who is 2 m tall is 79.2 in, or 6 ft, 7 in tall.

TABLE 4-4 Conversion from the Metric System to the U.S. Customary System

Convert from Metric System (Unit of 1)	Convert to U.S. System (Unit of 1)	Multiply by Conversion Factor
meter (m)	inch (in)	39.6 (1/0.0254)
meter (m)	yard (yd)	1.091 (1/0.91)
kilometer (km)	mile (mi)	0.621 (1/1.61)
gram (g)	ounce (oz)	0.035 (1/28.3)
kilogram (kg)	pound (lb)	2.21 or 2.2 (1/0.453)
milliliter (mL)	fluid ounce (fl oz)	0.034 (1/29.6)
milliliter (mL)	pint (pi)	2.11 (1/0.474)
liter (L)	gallon (gal)	0.264 (1/3.79)

If a patient weighs 55 kg, how many pounds does he weigh?

From Table 4-4, 1 kg is equal to 2.21 or 2.2 lb. To convert from kilograms to pounds, multiply the amount in kilograms by 2.2.

55 kg × 2.2 = 121

Therefore, 55 kg is equal to 121 lb.

If a patient voids 2.4 L of urine in a day, what is the amount in gallons?

The conversion factor between liters and gallons is 0.264. Therefore, multiply the amount in liters by 0.264 to arrive at the amount in gallons.

2.4 L × 0.264 = 0.63

Therefore, there are 0.63 gal in 2.4 L of urine.

Measurement of Temperature

The thermometers used in the clinical laboratory today originated in discoveries made by Galileo and others in the fifteenth and sixteenth centuries. Three types of measurement systems have evolved since then.

Fahrenheit Scale

Daniel Gabriel Fahrenheit invented the Fahrenheit scale for temperature measurement in 1724. He first used a mercury thermometer and a mixture of water, ice, and sal ammoniac to determine an artificial freezing point, which he designated as zero, and the boiling point of pure water (212°) as the upper point. Fahrenheit divided his thermometer into 212 equal parts. His final thermometer used the freezing point of water (32°) as the lower point and the temperature of the human body (96°) as the upper point. Soon after his death, the upper point of the Fahrenheit (F) scale was again moved to be 212°, while the freezing point remained unchanged and the thermometer was divided into 180 equal parts. The Fahrenheit system of measuring temperature is used by the general public in the United States.

Celsius Scale

In 1742 the Swedish astronomer Anders Celsius used the same fixed points of freezing and boiling water but set these points at 0 and 100, respectively. The thermometer was then divided into 100 equal parts. The Celsius, or Centigrade (C), system of temperature measurement is used by the public almost everywhere in the world, as well as by the scientific community.

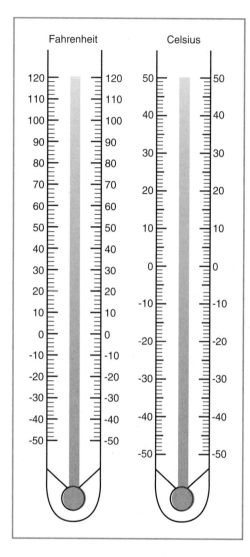

FIGURE 4-1 Fahrenheit versus Celsius thermometers. (From Doucette, L. J. [1997]. *Mathematics for the Clinical Laboratory* [p. 51]. Philadelphia: W.B. Saunders Company.)

Comparison of Temperature Scales

The Fahrenheit and Celsius temperature scales are shown in Figure 4-1. Note that the Celsius scale is divided into units of 10, while the Fahrenheit scale is quite different.

Conversion between Fahrenheit and Celsius Temperatures

Almost all temperatures in the clinical laboratory and many patient temperatures are taken using the Celsius scale. Therefore, it is helpful to be able to convert between Celsius and Fahrenheit temperatures. Note that the Fahrenheit scale is divided into 180 parts, while the Celsius scale is divided into 100 parts. The Fahrenheit degree is thus $\frac{9}{5}$ of the Celsius degree.

Conversion from Celsius to Fahrenheit

To convert from degrees Celsius to degrees Fahrenheit, remember that the Fahrenheit degree is $\frac{9}{5}$ of a Celsius degree because of the differences in their scales. Since 0°C is equal to 32°F, a factor of 32 must be included in the conversion in order to make the two scales equal. The following formula describes the relationship between Celsius and Fahrenheit temperatures:

$$°F = \frac{9}{5}°C + 32$$

or

$$°F = 1.8°C + 32$$

PROBLEMS

If a thermometer in the laboratory measured the temperature of a refrigerator at 3°C, what is the equivalent in degrees Fahrenheit?

To solve this problem, use the conversion formula:

$$°F = 1.8°C + 32$$

Substituting into the formula the Celsius temperature of the refrigerator, the following formula is derived:

$$°F = [(1.8)(°3)] + 32$$
$$= 5.4 + 32$$
$$= 37.4$$

Therefore, 3°C is equal to 37.4°F.

Convert 37°C to its equivalent in Fahrenheit.

Substituting into the formula to convert Celsius to Fahrenheit, the following equation is derived:

$$°F = [(1.8)(°37)] + 32$$
$$= 66.6 + 32$$
$$= 98.6$$

Therefore, 37°C is equivalent to 98.6°F.

Conversion from Fahrenheit to Celsius

To convert from Fahrenheit to Celsius, the above formula can be used backward. Since the two scales have different freezing temperatures (32° vs. 0°), the factor of 32 must first be subtracted from the Fahrenheit temperature. The product of this calculation is then multiplied by $\frac{5}{9}$.

PROBLEMS

If a thermometer reads 40°F, what is the equivalent in degrees Celsius?

To convert from Fahrenheit to Celsius, first subtract the factor of 32 from the Celsius temperature. Next, multiply the product of this calculation by 5/9.

The conversion formula from Fahrenheit to Celsius is:

$$°C = (°F - 32)\frac{5}{9}$$

Substituting the temperature of 40°F into the formula:

$$°C = (°40 - 32)\frac{5}{9}$$

$$= (8)\frac{5}{9}$$

$$= 4.4$$

Therefore, 40°F is equal to 4.4°C.

Convert 103°F to its equivalent in degrees Celsius.

Using the conversion formula, the following equation is derived:

$$°C = (°103 - 32)\frac{5}{9}$$

$$= (71)\frac{5}{9}$$

$$= 39.4$$

Therefore, 103°F is equivalent to 39.4°C.

EXAMPLE PROBLEMS

This section is designed to be useful to both the student and the health care practitioner. Students can use the example problems in order to master the material. The health care practitioner can use these problems as templates for solving calculations. Find an example problem similar to the problem that you need to solve and substitute into the equation the numbers appropriate to your calculation.

1. **Q Convert 200 pg to grams.**
   A 1 pg is equal to 1×10^{-12} g. Therefore, 200 pg is equal to 200×10^{-12} g or 2.00×10^{-10} g.

2. **Q How many milligrams are in 4.95 g?**

A There are 1000 mg in 1 g. Therefore, multiply 4.95 by 1000 to convert milligrams to grams: 4.95 × 1000 = 4950 mg.

3. **Q** **How many centimeters are there in 4 m?**

A There are 100 cm in 1 m. Therefore, there are 400 cm in 4 m.

4. **Q** **Express 4.5 mL in liters.**

A A milliliter is 1000 times smaller than a liter. To determine how many liters are in 4.5 mL, divide 4.5 by 1000: 4.5/1000 = 0.0045 or 4.5 × 10^{-3} L.

5. **Q** **How many meters are there in 100 yd?**

A One yard is slightly longer than 1 m. The conversion factor used to convert from yards to meters is 0.914. Multiply the amount in yards by 0.914 to convert to meters: 100 yd × 0.914 = 91.4 m.

6. **Q** **How many kilograms are there in 10 lb of dry weight?**

A To convert from pounds to kilograms, multiply the weight in pounds by the factor 0.453: 10 × 0.453 = 4.53 kg.

7. **Q** **A patient weighs 57 kg. How many pounds does the patient weigh?**

A To convert from kilograms to pounds, multiply the quantity in kilograms by 2.2: 57 × 2.2 = 125 lb.

8. **Q** **Convert 2.5 mg/mL to mg/L.**

A Use equivalent units to do this conversion. There are 1000 mL per liter, and 1000 mL/L is equivalent to 1. Therefore, we can use this fraction to cancel units and convert from mg/mL to mg/L.

$$\frac{2.5 \text{ mg}}{1 \text{ mL}} \times \frac{1000 \text{ mL}}{1 \text{ L}} = \frac{2500 \text{ mg}}{1 \text{ L}}$$

9. **Q** **Convert 250 mg/dL to g/L.**

A This is solved in two steps. First, convert milligrams to grams:

$$\frac{250 \text{ mg}}{1 \text{ dL}} \times \frac{1 \text{ g}}{1000 \text{ mg}} = \frac{0.250 \text{ g}}{1 \text{ dL}}$$

Next, convert deciliters to liters:

$$\frac{0.250 \text{ g}}{1 \text{ dL}} \times \frac{10 \text{ dL}}{1 \text{ L}} = \frac{2.50 \text{ g}}{1 \text{ L}}$$

10. **Q** **What is the Fahrenheit equivalent of 15°C?**

A The formula used to convert from Fahrenheit to Celsius is:

$$°F = \frac{9}{5}°C + 32$$

or

$$°F = 1.8°C + 32$$

Substituting into the formula the Celsius temperature:

$$°F = \frac{9}{5}15°C + 32$$
$$= 59.0.$$

11. **Q** **What is the Fahrenheit equivalent of −12°C?**

    A Use the formula:

    $$°F = 1.8°C + 32$$
    $$= (1.8)(-12°C) + 32$$
    $$= 10.4.$$

12. **Q** **What is the Celsius equivalent of 215°F?**

    A The formula used to convert from Celsius to Fahrenheit is:

    $$°C = (°F - 32)\frac{5}{9}$$

    Substituting into the formula the Fahrenheit temperature:

    $$°C = (215°F - 32)\frac{5}{9}$$
    $$= 101.7.$$

13. **Q** **What is the Celsius equivalent of −20°F?**

    A The formula used to convert from Celsius to Fahrenheit is:

    $$°C = (°F - 32)\frac{5}{9}$$

    Use the formula:

    $$°C = (-20°F - 32)\frac{5}{9}$$
    $$= -28.9.$$

PRACTICE PROBLEMS

Solve the following problems to further master the material. All answers and explanations to some problems can be found in a separate section at the back of the book.

Convert the following numbers to their metric equivalent.

1. 25.5 µg =   ? g
2. 30 mL =   ? L
3. 75 mm =   ? cm
4. 10 km =   ? m

 5. 1 L   =   ? dL
 6. 15 nm   =   ? mm
 7. 8 oz   =   ? g
 8. 72 in.   =   ? m
 9. 2 pt   =   ? mL
10. 1 gal   =   ? L

Convert:
11. 25 mg/dL to mg/L.
12. 4 mg/L to mg/dL.
13. 12 g/L to mg/dL.
14. 250 mg/dL to g/L.
15. 2 cm^2 to mm^2.

Convert:
16. 35°C to °F.
17. −4°C to °F.
18. 210°F to °C.
19. −5°F to °C.

CHAPTER 5

Dilutions and Titers

INTRODUCTION

This chapter introduces the reader to dilutions and titers. Many health care practitioners do not prepare dilutions or titers as part of their daily responsibilities, but they may have to work with medications diluted by other health care practitioners or understand vaccine titer reports from the clinical laboratory. Therefore, if you are a student in a health profession or a health care practitioner who does not deal with dilutions or titers, you may skip this chapter. Although this chapter contains more information than may be needed, there are health care practitioners who do require it.

Simple Dilutions

Preparing dilutions of medications or patient samples is an everyday activity in health care. Medications may have to be diluted in order to administer the prescribed dose to a patient, and in the clinical laboratory a specimen may have to be diluted in order to be analyzed. In chemistry, the specimen may have a concentration outside of the linear range of the method or instrument used for analysis. In microbiology, antibiotics are diluted to determine the minimum inhibitory concentration for microorganisms. Bleach is diluted to make a solution to clean and disinfect countertops, instruments, and patient examination rooms.

Serial dilutions are performed on serum in immunology to determine titers (or quantities) of antibodies. A poorly performed or interpreted dilution in the laboratory may lead to errors of analysis and may subsequently affect patient treatment. Even more important, a poorly performed dilution of therapeutic drugs may lead to medication errors that could directly harm patients, as they may be either over- or undermedicated.

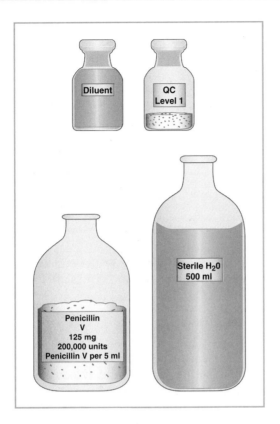

There are two parts to a dilution. The first part is the sample to be diluted; the second is the diluent used to perform the dilution. In the laboratory, many lyophilized or "freeze-dried" quality control materials have an accompanying diluent to be used for reconstitution. This diluent may contain buffers necessary to provide the correct concentration of the analytes to be tested. If deionized water is used instead of the manufacturer's supplied diluent, the control material will not be correctly buffered and inaccurate results may occur. Therefore, it is essential that the proper diluent be used for reconstitution.

Some medications come in powdered form and must be reconstituted before use. As with quality control material, it is important that the correct diluent and volume of diluent be used. In addition, once diluted, the medication must be given sufficient time to go completely into solution before being administered to the patient; otherwise, a lower than required dose may be given.

When a dilution is required, it is often referred to as a "1 to 10" ($^1/_{10}$) or a "1 to 2" ($^1/_2$) dilution. A 1 to 10 dilution means that for every 1 part of sample, there are 10 parts of solution. In a 1 to 10 dilution, 1 part of the sample and 9, *not* 10, parts of the diluent are used. If 10 parts of the diluent were used, there would be 11 parts to the solution.

A simple dilution uses the following formula:

$$\frac{SV}{SV + DV}$$

or

$$\frac{SV}{TV}$$

where

SV = sample volume
DV = diluent volume
TV = total volume

Note that the SV is included in the denominator of the equation. This is because it is part of the TV of the solution. Many dilution errors are made by forgetting this crucial fact.

PROBLEMS

 A 1 to 5 (⅕) dilution of serum is to be made on a sample that is too high to measure on the chemistry analyzer for the glucose method used. (When a result is too high to be measured by an instrument, the result is referred to as "outside of the linear range of the instrument.") The TV of the dilution is to be 100 μL. What volumes of serum and diluent (deionized water) are needed?

> **Note**   In this example, the instrument used to measure the glucose is not a glucose meter that uses whole blood, but rather an instrument that measures the glucose concentration in serum.

To solve this problem, use ratio and proportion:

$$\frac{1 \text{ part SV}}{5 \text{ parts TV}} = \frac{X \text{ parts SV}}{100 \text{ parts TV}}$$

(TV = 1 part SV + 4 parts DV)

Cross-multiplying the equation yields:

$$(1)(100) = (5)(X)$$
$$100 = 5X$$
$$20 = X$$

The SV is 20, and the DV is 100 − 20 or 80. This can be checked by reducing 20 and 80 by a factor of 20 to 1 and 4, or 1 part SV and 4 parts DV.

A 1 to 3 (⅓) dilution must be prepared to make a TV of 30 μL. How much sample must be used?

Again, use ratio and proportion to solve this problem:

$$\frac{1 \text{ part SV}}{3 \text{ parts TV}} = \frac{X \text{ parts SV}}{30 \text{ parts TV}}$$

Cross-multiplying the equation yields:

$$(1)(30.0) = (3)(X)$$
$$30 = 3X$$
$$10.0 = X$$

Therefore, 10 μL of sample and 20 μL of diluent will be used for the dilution.

A pharmacist must prepare a 1 to 10 (¹⁄₁₀) dilution of a stock drug for a pediatric patient. The total volume is 5 mL. How much of the drug and how much diluent must be used to make this dilution?

Using ratio and proportion:

$$\frac{1 \text{ part SV}}{10 \text{ parts TV}} = \frac{X \text{ parts SV}}{5 \text{ parts TV}}$$

Cross-multiplying the equation yields:

$$(1)(5.0) = (10)(X)$$
$$5.0 = 10 \, X$$
$$0.5 \text{ mL} = X$$

Therefore, 0.5 mL of sample will be used for the dilution.

Since TV = SV + DV, the amount of DV is:

$$5.0 \, (TV) - 0.5 \, (SV) = X \, DV$$
$$4.5 \text{ mL} = DV$$

Therefore, 0.5 mL of the drug must be used and diluted with 4.5 mL of diluent to make the 1 to 10 (¹⁄₁₀) dilution for the pediatric patient.

In the laboratory, once a specimen has been diluted and analyzed, the result obtained *must be corrected for the dilution*. A common preventable laboratory error is the failure to correct a diluted specimen's result. An easy way to correct the result is to use a factor. This factor is the reciprocal of the dilution that was performed. In the first example, a 1 to 5 (⅕) dilution was performed. The factor for this dilution is the reciprocal of 1 to 5 (⅕), or 5.

$$1 \div \frac{1}{5} \quad \text{or} \quad \frac{1}{\frac{1}{5}} = 5$$

The glucose result obtained from the first example would be multiplied by 5 to obtain its true value.

Using the glucose example, suppose that the linear range of the glucose assay that could be measured by the instrument is 25 to 600 mg/dL. A patient sample is analyzed, and the result is too high to be measured by the instrument. A 1 to 5 ($\frac{1}{5}$) dilution is performed on the serum, and the reanalyzed diluted sample result is 130 mg/dL. The diluted sample result must be multiplied by the dilution factor to determine the concentration in the undiluted sample.

130 mg/dL × 5 (dilution factor) = 650 mg/dL

Therefore, the patient's actual glucose result is 650 mg/dL, *not* 130 mg/dL. Failure to perform this crucial step would mean reporting a glucose level of 130 mg/dL instead of 650 mg/dL, a misdiagnosis that could have major effects on the health of the patient.

PROBLEM

A patient's cholesterol result is outside the linear range of the analyzer, so 10 μL of serum is added to 90 μL of diluent and the diluted sample is reanalyzed. The cholesterol value of the diluted sample is 45 mg/dL. What cholesterol value is reported to the physician and/or placed in the patient's chart, and what is the dilution factor that will be used to calculate this result?

The first step is to determine the dilution that was performed:

$$\frac{10\ \mu L}{10\ \mu L + 90\ \mu L} = \frac{10}{100} = \frac{1}{10}$$

Next, the dilution factor is the reciprocal of the dilution that was performed, in this case 1 to 10.

$$\text{Dilution factor} = 1 \div \frac{1}{10} \quad \text{or} \quad \frac{1}{\frac{1}{10}} = 10$$

The last step is to multiply the diluted result by the factor:

45 mg/dL × 10 = 450 mg/dL

The health care practitioner reports a cholesterol value of 450 mg/dL to the physician. This example demonstrates how critical it is to perform the dilution calculations correctly. In this example, a cholesterol value of 45 mg/dL is abnormally low, and a value of 450 mg/dL is abnormally high.

Dilutions versus Ratios

Dilutions and ratios can be confusing for students because different textbooks refer to them in different ways. In this book, dilutions will be designated by a slash, as in ½, and ratios will be designated by a colon, as in 1:4. In a ratio, the numerator is the parts of the sample used, and the denominator is the parts or amounts of diluent used.

Ratio: 1:4 = 1 part sample, 4 parts diluent

Contrast this with a dilution in which the numerator denotes the parts of the sample used but the denominator is the *total number of parts* (diluent plus the sample).

Dilution: ¼ = 1 part sample, 3 parts diluent

In the above ratio example, a 1:4 ratio is a ⅕ dilution.

Another way of stating the difference between ratios and dilutions is that a *dilution* is formed by the *ratio* of the SV to the TV. The ratio tells you how much of the sample and diluent are necessary to form the dilution. Using the above example, the 1:4 ratio indicates that you need 1 part sample to 4 parts diluent in order to make a ⅕ dilution.

PROBLEM

To clarify the difference between a ratio and a dilution, suppose that 25 µL of serum is added to 100 µL of diluent. What is the ratio of serum to diluent? What is the dilution in this example?

The ratio of serum to diluent is 25 parts serum to 100 parts diluent, or a 1:4 ratio. In this example, 25 parts of serum were diluted into 100 parts of diluent. Using the dilution formula:

$$\frac{25 \ \mu L \ (SV)}{25 \ \mu L \ (SV) + 100 \ \mu L \ (DV)}$$

$$= \frac{25 \ \mu L \ (SV)}{125 \ \mu L \ (TV)}$$

$$= \frac{1}{5}$$

Therefore, 25 parts of sample to 100 parts of diluent is a 1:4 *ratio* but a ⅕ *dilution*. This distinction is critical when calculating the original concentration.

Serial Dilutions and Multiple Dilutions

Often in immunology or microbiology, serial dilutions are performed. An advantage of a serial dilution is that very large dilutions of serum can occur with only a small amount of serum and diluent used. For example, suppose that a ¹/₁₀₀₀ dilution of serum is needed for a test. Theoretically, 1.0 mL of sample and 999.0 mL of diluent could be used (or 0.5 mL of sample and 499.5 mL of diluent). However, these are large volumes of diluent and sample. Using serial dilutions, much smaller sample and diluent volumes can be used. A serial dilution is simply a series of sequential dilutions of the sample until the final dilution is reached. By definition, a serial dilution uses the same dilution for each tube in the series. A multiple dilution series uses different dilutions for each tube. In both cases, the final dilution is the sum product of each individual dilution:

Final dilution = (dilution 1)(dilution 2)(dilution 3) etc.

In immunology, serial dilutions are performed using the same dilution over and over again. If a serial dilution is composed of a series of $^1/_{10}$ dilutions, that dilution series can be referred to as a *10-fold* dilution series. Common serial dilutions series used in immunology are $^1/_2$, $^1/_4$, and $^1/_{10}$. If reagents are to be added directly to serially diluted tubes, it is important to discard from the last tube in the series the same sample volume used for all other dilutions in the series. For example, if a 10-fold dilution was performed with five tubes with an SV of 10 μL and a DV of 90 μL, 10 μL from the fifth tube must be discarded. If the 10 μL is not removed from the last tube, its TV will be 100 μL. However, all of the other tubes have a TV of 90 μL, since 10 μL is removed from each tube to be used in the next dilution in the series. By removing 10 μL from the last tube, when additional reagents are added to the diluted tubes, all tubes in the reaction sequence will have the same volume.

For clinical chemistry analyses, samples may be serially diluted or multiple dilution series may be used. In both cases, if the original concentration is known, the concentration of each tube in the series can be calculated in one of two ways.

A multiple dilution is performed on a sample to check the pipetting skills of a student technologist. Five tubes are used in the dilution. The concentration of the sample is 1500 mg/dL. The sample is diluted $^1/_5$ (tube 1), rediluted $^1/_2$ (tube 2), diluted again $^1/_4$ (tube 3), then $^1/_5$ (tube 4), and then $^1/_{10}$ (tube 5). After the student performs the dilution, the diluted specimen will be analyzed and the student will be graded on the precision of pipetting. What will be the diluted concentration in each tube? Figure 5-1 is a schematic of the multiple dilution.

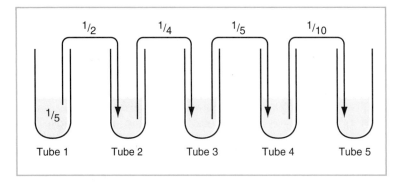

FIGURE 5-1 Schematic of multiple dilutions. (From Doucette, L. J. [1997]. *Mathematics for the Clinical Laboratory* [p. 66]. Philadelphia: W.B. Saunders.)

Method 1 to Determine the Concentration of Each Tube

1. Divide the first tube in the series by the dilution factor used in its dilution ($\frac{1}{5}$ dilution was performed; therefore, factor = 5). The sample concentration in tube 1 is:

$$\frac{1500 \text{ mg/dL}}{5} \quad \text{or} \quad 300 \text{ mg/dL}$$

2. Divide the concentration of the first tube by the dilution performed for the second tube (dilution was $\frac{1}{2}$; therefore, factor = 2). The concentration of tube 2 is:

$$\frac{300 \text{ mg/dL}}{2} \quad \text{or} \quad 150 \text{ mg/dL}$$

3. Divide the concentration of the second tube by the dilution performed for the third tube (dilution was $\frac{1}{4}$; therefore, factor = 4). Tube 3's concentration is:

$$\frac{150 \text{ mg/dL}}{4} \quad \text{or} \quad 37.5 \text{ mg/dL}$$

4. Divide the concentration of the third tube by the dilution performed for the fourth tube (dilution was $\frac{1}{5}$; therefore, factor = 5). Tube 4's concentration is:

$$\frac{37.5}{5} \quad \text{or} \quad 7.5 \text{ mg/dL}$$

5. Divide the concentration of tube 4 by the dilution performed for tube 5 (dilution was $\frac{1}{10}$; therefore, factor = 10). Tube 5 has a concentration of:

$$\frac{7.5}{10} \quad \text{or} \quad 0.75 \text{ mg/dL}$$

Method 2 to Determine the Concentration of Each Tube

1. Divide the original concentration by the dilution *factor* used for tube 1 to determine the concentration of tube 1.

$$\frac{1500}{5} = 300 \text{ mg/dL}$$

2. Determine the dilution, and therefore the dilution factor, for tube 2 by multiplying the dilutions performed on tube 1 and tube 2.

$$\frac{1}{5} \quad \times \quad \frac{1}{2} \quad = \quad \frac{1}{10}$$

Tube 1　　Tube 2　　Dilution for tube 2

Dilution factor = 10

Divide the original concentration by the dilution factor for tube 2.

$$\frac{1500}{10} = 150 \text{ mg/dL}$$

3. Determine the dilution, and therefore the dilution factor, for tube 3 by multiplying the dilutions performed on tubes 1, 2, and 3.

$$\frac{1}{5} \quad \times \quad \frac{1}{2} \quad \times \quad \frac{1}{4} \quad = \quad \frac{1}{40}$$

Tube 1   Tube 2   Tube 3   Dilution for tube 3

Dilution factor = 40

Or multiply the dilution of tube 2 by the dilution performed on tube 3.

$$\frac{1}{10} \times \frac{1}{4} = \frac{1}{40}$$

Divide the original concentration by the dilution factor for tube 3.

$$\frac{1500}{40} = 37.5 \text{ mg/dL}$$

4. Determine the dilution, and the dilution factor, for tube 4 by multiplying the dilutions performed on tubes 1, 2, 3, and 4.

$$\frac{1}{5} \quad \times \quad \frac{1}{2} \quad \times \quad \frac{1}{4} \quad \times \quad \frac{1}{5} \quad = \quad \frac{1}{200}$$

Tube 1   Tube 2   Tube 3   Tube 4   Dilution for tube 4

Dilution factor = 200

Or multiply the dilution of tube 3 by the dilution performed on tube 4.

$$\frac{1}{40} \times \frac{1}{5} = \frac{1}{200}$$

Divide the original concentration by the dilution factor for tube 4.

$$\frac{1500}{200} = 7.5 \text{ mg/dL}$$

5. Determine the dilution, and the dilution factor, for tube 5 by multiplying the dilutions performed on tubes 1, 2, 3, 4, and 5.

$$\frac{1}{5} \quad \times \quad \frac{1}{2} \quad \times \quad \frac{1}{4} \quad \times \quad \frac{1}{5} \quad \times \quad \frac{1}{10} \quad = \quad \frac{1}{2000}$$

Tube 1   Tube 2   Tube 3   Tube 4   Tube 5   Dilution for tube 5

Dilution factor = 2000

Or multiply the dilution of tube 4 by the dilution performed on tube 5.

$$\frac{1}{200} \times \frac{1}{10} = \frac{1}{2000}$$

Divide the original concentration by the dilution factor for tube 5.

$$\frac{1500}{2000} = 0.75 \text{ mg/dL}$$

To check this result, multiply 1500 by the product of the individual dilutions.

$(1500)(\frac{1}{5} \times \frac{1}{2} \times \frac{1}{4} \times \frac{1}{5} \times \frac{1}{10}) = (1500)(\frac{1}{2000}) = 0.75 \text{ mg/dL}$

Any of the dilutions performed in a serial or multiple dilution can be re-checked in this manner to verify the accuracy of the calculations that were performed.

Usually, serial dilutions are performed as a method of diluting a sample using the smallest quantities of sample and diluent possible. In the laboratory, how a dilution is performed is often limited by the types of pipettes available. Often the volumes of the available pipettes are used as the base from which the dilutions are calculated. It does not make sense to calculate a dilution in which 5 µL of sample is required when the smallest volume pipette available is 10 µL.

PROBLEMS

 A ¹/₁₀₀₀ dilution of a serum sample must be made. How is this done using small volumes of serum and diluent?

Perform a serial dilution on the serum specimen. Figure 5-2 is a schematic of the dilution.

Step 1.   Perform a ¹/₁₀ dilution of the serum (10 µL of serum to 90 µL of diluent) (tube 1).

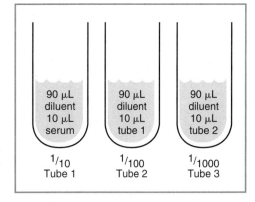

FIGURE 5-2   Schematic of a ¹/₁₀₀₀ serial dilution. (From Doucette, L. J. [1997]. *Mathematics for the Clinical Laboratory* [p. 69]. Philadelphia: W.B. Saunders.)

Step 2. Perform a $\frac{1}{10}$ dilution of tube 1 (10 µL in tube 1 to 90 µL of diluent in tube 2) (tube 2).

Step 3. Perform a $\frac{1}{10}$ dilution of tube 2 (10 µL in tube 1 to 90 µL of diluent in tube 3) (tube 3).

Tube 1 is diluted $\frac{1}{10}$

Tube 2 is diluted $\frac{1}{100}$:

$$\frac{1}{10} \times \frac{1}{10} = \frac{1}{100}$$

Tube 3 is diluted $\frac{1}{1000}$:

$$\frac{1}{100} \times \frac{1}{10} = \frac{1}{1000}$$

Thus, only 10 µL of sample and 270 µL of diluent are required to make the $\frac{1}{1000}$ dilution.

In immunology, serial dilutions of serum samples are often made. How can a final dilution of $\frac{1}{320}$ be made?

The first step is to determine the serial dilution scheme. Two questions to consider are What dilutions should be made? and How many dilutions are necessary? Common serial dilution schemes use a factor of 2, 4, 5, or 10 to make the serial dilutions. A $\frac{1}{320}$ dilution can be made in a number of ways. A $\frac{1}{2}$ serial dilution can be made to a final concentration of $\frac{1}{32}$ followed by a $\frac{1}{10}$ dilution ($\frac{1}{2} \rightarrow \frac{1}{4} \rightarrow \frac{1}{8} \rightarrow \frac{1}{16} \rightarrow \frac{1}{32}$, then $\frac{1}{10}$ of the $\frac{1}{32}$ dilution). Alternatively, the dilution scheme can be increased by a factor of 10 from the start. Figure 5-3 demonstrates this serial dilution scheme. The dilution is made starting with a $\frac{1}{20}$ dilution followed by a series of $\frac{1}{2}$ serial dilutions. *Note:* All tubes must be well mixed before sampling for the subsequent tube.

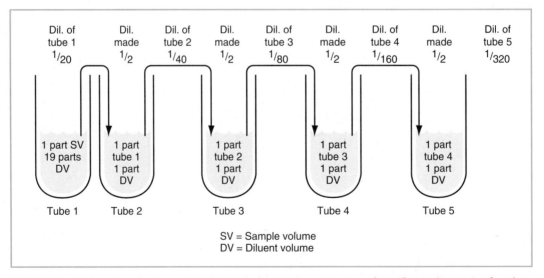

FIGURE 5-3 Schematic of a $\frac{1}{320}$ serial dilution. (From Doucette, L. J. [1997]. *Mathematics for the Clinical Laboratory* [p. 70]. Philadelphia: W.B. Saunders.)

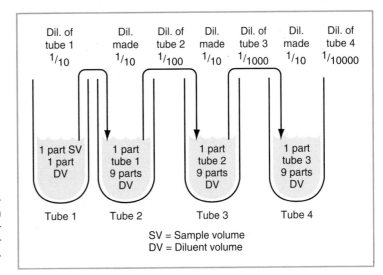

FIGURE 5-4 Schematic of a 10-fold serial dilution. (From Doucette, L. J. [1997]. *Mathematics for the Clinical Laboratory* [p. 70]. Philadelphia: W.B. Saunders.)

Some common serial dilution protocols used in the clinical laboratory are shown in Figures 5-4 to 5-6.

Titers

In immunology, *titers* are measured to determine the quantity of antibody present in a patient's sample. Sometimes this information is used to determine the patient's level of protective antibodies against disease, as in rubella or mumps. At

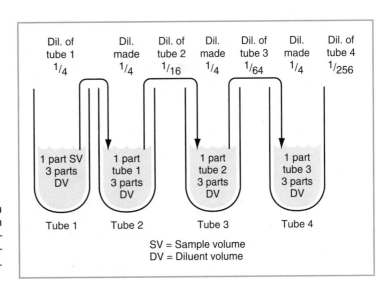

FIGURE 5-5 Schematic of a fourfold serial dilution. (From Doucette, L. J. [1997]. *Mathematics for the Clinical Laboratory* [p. 71]. Philadelphia: W.B. Saunders.)

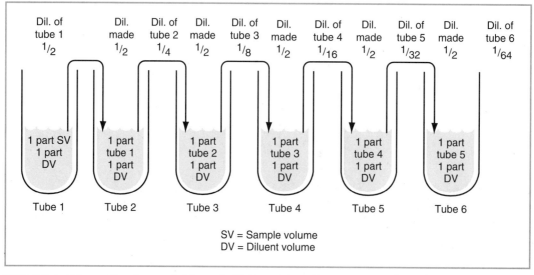

FIGURE 5-6 Schematic of a twofold serial dilution. (From Doucette, L. J. [1997]. *Mathematics for the Clinical Laboratory* [p. 71]. Philadelphia: W.B. Saunders.)

other times, it is used to determine the concentration of antibodies that leads to disease, such as the level of autoantibodies present in the patient's serum. A titer is the inverse of the dilution used in which a reaction occurs when antigen-antibody interactions are tested. A low titer of a protective antibody may mean that the patient does not have immunity to the disease being tested. When a titer analysis is performed, serial dilutions of the patient's serum are made in individual test tubes or wells, and antigen is added to each tube or well. The dilution in which the last measurable reaction occurs is the dilution used as the titer.

PROBLEMS

A rubella titer analysis is performed on a pregnant patient. Serial dilutions of the patient's serum are made at 1/20, 1/40, 1/80, 1/160, 1/320, 1/640, and 1/1280. Rubella antigen is added to each tube. A positive reaction is found in all but the 1/1280 dilution. What is the patient's titer?

The patient's rubella titer is 640 since the last positive reaction occurred at the 1/640 dilution.

An infectious mononucleosis antibody titer analysis is performed on a 16-year-old boy. A fourfold dilution series is positive at the 1/4, 1/16, and 1/64 dilutions but negative at the 1/256 dilution. What is the boy's antibody titer?

Since the last positive dilution was 1/64, the patient's antibody titer is 64.

EXAMPLE PROBLEMS

This section is designed to be useful to both the student and the health care practitioner. Students can use the example problems in order to master the material. The health care practitioner can use these problems as templates for performing laboratory calculations. Find an example problem similar to the problem that you need to solve and substitute into the equation the numbers appropriate to your calculation.

1. **Q In a ¹/₅ dilution, how many parts of diluent are needed?**

   A A ¹/₅ dilution consists of 1 part sample to 4 parts diluent. This is because the *total* volume is 5 parts (1 part sample + 4 parts diluent). This is expressed mathematically as:

   $$\frac{SV}{SV + DV}$$

   or

   $$\frac{SV}{TV}$$

2. **Q If 1 mL of sample is added to 4 mL of diluent, what is the dilution factor?**

   A The dilution factor is the reciprocal of the dilution. In this question, 1 mL of sample is added to 4 mL of diluent. The dilution performed can be calculated by using the formula in example problem 1. The dilution is a ¹/₅ dilution (1 part SV to 5 parts TV). Therefore, the dilution factor is the reciprocal of ¹/₅, or 5.0.

3. **Q A serum sample is outside the linear range of the analyzer for an analyte. A 1:2 ratio of serum to diluent is obtained, and the sample is reanalyzed. What factor would be needed to multiply the result of the diluted sample in order to obtain the correct concentration of the analyte?**

   A A 1:2 ratio is 1 part sample to 2 parts diluent. This is exactly the same as a ¹/₃ dilution. The diluted result must be multiplied by 3, not 2, to obtain a correct result.

4. **Q A ¹/₁₀ dilution is to be performed on a sample. A serum volume of 100 μL is available for the dilution, but the medical assistant cannot use all of it because a repeat analysis may be necessary. How should the dilution be performed?**

A To determine the SV necessary, divide the TV of serum by the dilution factor of 10. Remember, the dilution factor is the reciprocal of the dilution. This yields an SV of 10 µL and leaves 90 µL of serum available for further testing.

5. **Q** **A serum triglyceride sample is diluted ¹/₁₀, with a result of 75 mg/dL. What is the patient's actual triglyceride level?**

   A Since the sample is diluted ¹/₁₀, the diluted result must be multiplied by the dilution factor. This dilution factor is the reciprocal of the dilution performed. In this problem, since a ¹/₁₀ dilution is performed, the dilution factor is 10. Therefore, the result of 75 mg/dL is multiplied by 10 to yield the actual result of 750 mg/dL.

6. **Q** **In a multiple dilution series, 15 µL of serum and 60 µL of diluent are added and mixed in tube 1. From tube 1, 10 µL is taken and placed in 40 µL of diluent in tube 2. What is the final dilution in tube 2?**

   A The final dilution is the product of the individual dilutions in the multiple dilution series. The first dilution is a ¹/₅ dilution since 15 µL of sample is added to a TV of 75 µL ($^{15}/_{75}$ = ¹/₅). The second dilution is also ¹/₅, as 10 µL of serum is added to a TV of 50 µL ($^{10}/_{50}$ = ¹/₅). Therefore, the final dilution is:

   $$\text{Final dilution} = \frac{1}{5} \times \frac{1}{5} = \frac{1}{25}$$

   The sample in tube 2 is diluted ¹/₂₅.

7. **Q** **Using the dilution from example problem 6, if the original concentration of the sample was 150 mg/dL, what is the concentration of the sample in tube 1?**

   A To determine the concentration of the first tube in a serial or multiple dilution series, divide the sample concentration in the first tube in the series by the dilution factor used in its dilution. In this case, 150 mg/dL is divided by the factor of 5 since a ¹/₅ dilution was performed in tube 1. This yields a concentration of 30 mg/dL in tube 1.

8. **Q** **A 10-fold serial dilution is performed, with a final dilution of ¹/₁₀,₀₀₀. The first dilution in the series in tube 1 is ¹/₁₀. If the original concentration had been 35,000 ng/dL, what would the concentration be in tube 4?**

   A A 10-fold serial dilution means that each tube in the series is diluted ¹/₁₀. Therefore, the first tube is diluted ¹/₁₀, and the second is diluted ¹/₁₀ with the SV coming from tube 1. The third tube is also diluted ¹/₁₀, with its SV coming from the diluted tube 2. The dilutions and concentrations in each tube can be calculated in two different ways. The first method calculates the concentration in each tube by dividing each tube by its dilution factor. For example, tube 1 is diluted $^1/_{10}$. If the original concentration is 35,000 ng/mL, the concentration in tube 1 is $^{35,000}/_{10}$ or 3500. The concentration in tube 2 can be calculated by dividing the concentration in tube 1 by the dilution performed in tube 2. In this case, $^{3500}/_{10} = 350$. The concentration in tube 3 can be calculated by dividing the concentration in tube 2 by the dilution factor of 10 as well; $^{350}/_{10} = 35$. The concentration in tube 4 can be calculated by dividing the concentration in tube 3 by the dilution factor of 10. Therefore, the concentration in tube 4 is 3.5 ng/mL.

The second method used to determine the concentration in each tube in a series is to multiply the individual dilutions performed on the previous tubes and divide the original concentration by the product of the individual dilutions. For example, tube 1 is a $^1/_{10}$ dilution, tube 2 is a $^1/_{10}$ dilution, tube 3 is a $^1/_{10}$ dilution, and tube 4 is a $^1/_{10}$ dilution. Therefore, in tube 4, the dilution is:

$$\frac{1}{10} \times \frac{1}{10} \times \frac{1}{10} \times \frac{1}{10} = \frac{1}{10,000}$$

In tube 4, a $^1/_{10,000}$ dilution was performed. By dividing the original concentration by 10,000, the concentration in tube 4 can be calculated:

$$\frac{35,000}{10,000} = 3.5 \text{ ng/mL.}$$

Therefore, both methods yield the same result: a concentration of 75 ng/mL in tube 3.

9. Q **If a serial dilution is performed and a final concentration of the sample is 0.296 mg/dL, with a dilution factor of 1200, what is the original concentration?**

A To determine the original concentration, multiply the dilution factor by the final diluted sample. In this case, 1200 × 0.296 mg/dL = 355.2 mg/dL. The original concentration is 355.2 mg/dL.

10. Q **A multiple dilution series is performed to determine the antistreptolysin O titer of a patient. The multiple dilution series consisted of $^1/_{100}$, $^1/_{125}$, $^1/_{166}$, $^1/_{250}$, $^1/_{500}$, $^1/_{625}$, $^1/_{833}$, and $^1/_{1250}$ dilutions of the patient's serum. One milliliter of each dilution is added to the test tubes. Streptolysin antigen is added to all tubes and incubated, and streptolysin O cells are then added. The presence of the strep-**

tolysin O antibody in the patient's serum binds the streptolysin antigen and prevents hemolysis of the O cells. The $1/250$ dilution tube is the first tube to exhibit hemolysis. What is the patient's titer?

A The last dilution tube not to exhibit hemolysis, or to demonstrate a positive reaction, is the tube with the $1/166$ dilution. Therefore, the patient's titer is 166 Todd units.

PRACTICE PROBLEMS

Solve the following practice problems to further master the material. All answers and explanations to some problems can be found in a separate section at the back of the book.

Calculate the dilution factors for the following problems.
1. 4 mL of sample added to 12 mL of diluent
2. 0.5 mL of sample added to 2 mL of diluent
3. 10 µL of sample added to 190 µL of diluent
4. 20 µL of sample added to 80 µL of diluent

Use the following information to answer questions 5–8. A multiple dilution series was performed. The sample was diluted $1/2$, $1/2$, and $1/4$.
5. What is the final dilution?
6. What is the final dilution factor?
7. What is the concentration in tube 2 if the original concentration was 100?
8. What is the dilution factor for tube 1?
9. A cytomegalovirus (CMV) antibody titer test was performed on a 2-week-old infant. The serum was tested with CMV antigen in the following sequence: undiluted and diluted $1/2$, $1/4$, $1/8$, and $1/16$. Positive reactions were noted in the undiluted, $1/2$, $1/4$, and $1/8$ tubes. What is the baby's CMV antibody titer?
10. An antithyroid microsomal antibody test was performed on a 45-year-old man. The dilution sequence was performed in a microtiter plate by first adding 25 µL of serum to 100 µL of diluent in well 1. Then 25 µL of the first dilution was added to 100 µL of the diluent in well 2. Next, 25 µL from well 2 was added to 75 µL of the diluent in well 3. Wells 4 through 12 were serially diluted in a fourfold dilution series. What would the dilution be in well 6?

CHAPTER 6

Calculations Associated with Solutions

Upon completion of this chapter, the reader should be able to:

1. Perform calculations to determine percent weight/volume (% w/v), percent volume/volume (% v/v) or percent weight/weight (% w/w) concentrations of solutions.

2. Perform ratio and proportion calculations to determine the concentration of solutes and solvents.

INTRODUCTION

This chapter introduces the reader to solutions. Many health care practitioners do not make solutions as part of their daily responsibilities, but they may have to work with solutions prepared by other health care practitioners. One common solution used in health care is bleach solution, and all medications given by intravenous route are contained within a solution. However, if you are a student in a health profession or a health care practitioner who does not deal with solutions, you may skip this chapter. Although this chapter contains more information than may be needed, there are health care practitioners who do require it.

Percent Solutions

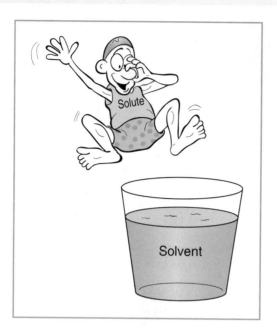

Solutions are used in the clinical laboratory and for certain liquid and semisolid medications. They consist of a *solute* and a *solvent*. The solute is the chemical or medication that is dissolved in the solution, and the solvent is the liquid or semisolid material in which the solute is dissolved. In the clinical laboratory, the solvent may be deionized water, physiologic saline, or a specific diluent. For medications, it may be sterile water, physiologic saline, or, for semisolid medications such as creams and ointments, some type of base cream. There are three types of percent solutions: percent weight/weight, percent weight/volume, and percent volume/volume. In all three types, the total volume of the solvent is 100 mL.

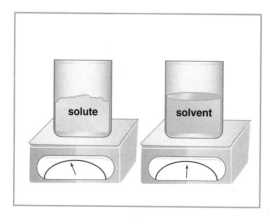

Percent Weight/Weight (% w/w)

A % w/w solution is calculated by the following formula:

$$\% \text{ w/w} = \frac{\text{gram of solute}}{100 \text{ g of solution}} \quad \text{or} \quad \text{gram of solute per 100 g of solution}$$

In this type of solution, the amounts of solute and solvent are *weighed* individually using a balance. Note that since the total is based on 100 g of *solution*, the amount of solvent that must be weighed is determined by subtracting the quantity of solute needed from 100. Once the amount of solvent is determined, the solvent and solute are mixed together in a flask or beaker. The % w/w solutions are the most accurate because, unlike percent weight/volume (% w/v) solutions, their measurements do not fluctuate with temperature. Pharmacists, chemists, and other research scientists may use the % w/w method to make solutions, but otherwise it is not commonly used.

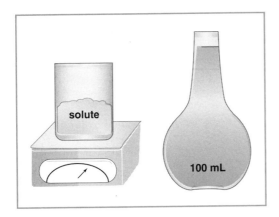

Percent Weight/Volume (% w/v)

A % w/v solution is calculated by the following formula:

$$\% \text{ w/v} = \frac{\text{gram of solute}}{100 \text{ mL of solution}} \quad \text{or} \quad \text{gram of solute per 100 mL of solution}$$

The % w/v solution is the most frequently used percent solution in the clinical laboratory and for medications. Pharmacists frequently use this type of solution to make elixirs or other liquid solutions. In this type of solution, the amount of solute is weighed on a balance and then placed in a 100 mL volumetric flask containing a small amount of solvent to dissolve the solute. Once the solute is dissolved, the remaining solvent is added to the volumetric flask to the calibrated mark. The term *quantity sufficient* (*qs*) is often used in the laboratory to describe the addition of the solvent to the calibrated mark. For example, you may be instructed to add a determined amount of solute to a volumetric flask and then qs it to the calibration mark with the appropriate solvent.

Many medications use a total volume that is less than 100 mL, and the amount of diluent to be used is stated on the label. A standard pharmaceutical medication concentration is X mg of drug/5 mL; that is, for every 5 mL (or 1 teaspoon) of liquid medication, there are X mg of the drug. However, some medications have concentrations of X mg drug/mL in a vial or another container that holds a total volume of 5 mL. Giving 5 mL of this type of drug would mean giving a dose five times the prescribed concentration. Therefore, it is *imperative* that all medication labels be carefully read and the dosage requirements understood prior to dispensing the medication to the patient.

PROBLEMS

What is the % w/v of a solution that has 2500 mg (or 2.5 g) of penicillin V dissolved in a total volume of 100 mL of deionized water?

To solve this problem, use the formula for % w/v:

$$X \text{ \% w/v} = \frac{2.5 \text{ g penicillin V}}{100 \text{ mL of solution}}$$

$$X = 0.025\% \text{ w/v}$$

Therefore, a solution with 2500 mg of penicillin V dissolved in 100 mL of water has a % w/v concentration of 0.025%.

What is the % w/v of a solution that has 900 mg of sodium chloride (NaCl) dissolved in 100 mL of deionized water?

Remember, the % w/v formula is based on grams per 100 mL of solution. Therefore, the first step is to convert the 900 mg into grams, or 0.9 g. Next, substitute the known values into the % w/v equation:

$$X \text{ \% w/v} = \frac{0.9 \text{ g NaCl}}{100 \text{ mL of solution}}$$

$$X = 0.9\% \text{ w/v}$$

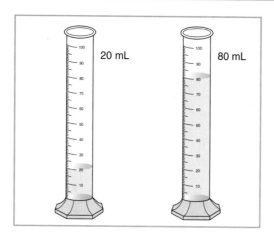

20 mL

80 mL

Percent Volume/Volume (% v/v)

A % v/v solution is calculated by the following formula:

$$\% \text{ v/v} = \frac{\text{mL of solute}}{100 \text{ mL of solution}} \quad \text{or} \quad \text{mL of solute per 100 mL of solution}$$

The % v/v measure is similar to % w/w in that the *total* volume of the solution is 100 mL. Therefore, the amount of solvent is determined by the following formula:

100 mL total volume − amount of solute = amount of solvent

PROBLEM

How many milliliters of ethanol (EtOH) are needed to make a 75% v/v solution using deionized water as the solvent?

Using the formula for % v/v and substituting in the appropriate given numbers, the following equation is derived:

75% v/v EtOH = X mL of EtOH in 100 mL of solution

X = 75 mL of EtOH

How many milliliters of water are necessary for this solution?

The amount of water needed is determined by the formula:

Amount of solvent = 100 − amount of solute

X = 100 − 75

X = 25

Therefore, 75 mL of EtOH would be added to 25 mL of deionized water to produce a solution of 75% v/v of EtOH.

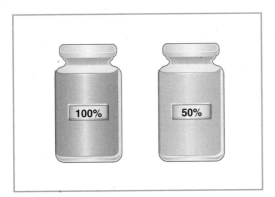

Concentration Calculations

Sometimes in the clinical laboratory or in a health care environment, a concentrated solution, called the *stock solution*, must be diluted to make a less concentrated solution. The following formula can be used whenever a calculation involves changing concentrations between two solutions:

$$C_1V_1 = C_2V_2$$

where:

C_1 = stock concentration
V_1 = volume of stock required
C_2 = concentration of the new solution
V_2 = volume of the new solution

Because this is a derivation of a ratio and proportion formula, if three of the four amounts are known, the fourth amount can be calculated.

PROBLEMS

A total volume of 300 mL of a 10% w/v bleach solution are needed. In the stockroom is a bottle of laundry bleach (although technically not true, assume a 100% w/v concentration). How many milliliters of the stock bleach solution are necessary to make the 10% w/v solution?

Using the formula for concentrations, the following equation can be derived:

$$C_1V_1 = C_2V_2$$

where:

C_1 = 100% w/v
V_1 = X
C_2 = 10% w/v
V_2 = 300 mL

As long as the same units are used on both sides of the equation, units do not have to be included in the equation.

$$(100.0)(X) = (10)(300)$$
$$= 3000$$
$$X = 30 \text{ mL}$$

Therefore, 30 mL of the 100% w/v solution are diluted with water (or qs) to a total volume of 300 mL.

The directions for a new 10% stock sterilizing solution call for it to be diluted to a 2% solution before use. How should the medical assistant perform this dilution?

The medical assistant can use the concentration formula to perform the dilution and use a total volume of 100 mL to make the math calculations easier. Using the concentration formula:

$$C_1V_1 = C_2V_2$$

where:

$$C_1 = 10\%$$
$$V_1 = X \text{ mL}$$
$$C_2 = 2\%$$
$$V_2 = 100 \text{ mL}$$
$$(10)(X) = (2.0)(100)$$
$$10X = 200$$
$$X = \frac{200}{10}$$
$$= 20$$

The medical assistant would use 20 mL of the stock sterilizing solution and add 80 mL of sterile water to make a total concentration of 100 mL of a 2% sterilizing solution.

In this problem, 250 mL of a stock sodium hydroxide (NaOH) solution is placed in a volummetric flask and diluted to a total volume of 1 L. The concentration of the diluted specimen is 1.00 Molar (M). What is the concentration of the stock NaOH?

Using the concentration formula:

$$C_1V_1 = C_2V_2$$

where:

$$C_1 = X$$
$$V_1 = 250 \text{ mL}$$
$$C_2 = 1 \text{ M}$$
$$V_2 = 1000 \text{ mL}$$
$$(X)(250) = (1)(1000)$$
$$(250)(X) = 1000$$
$$X = 4$$

Therefore, the stock solution has a concentration of 4 M.

EXAMPLE PROBLEMS

This section is designed to be useful to both the student and the health care practitioner. Students can use the example problems in order to master the material. The health care practitioner can use these problems as templates for solving calculations. Find an example problem similar to the problem that you need to solve and substitute into the equation the numbers appropriate to your calculation.

1. **Q How is 100 mL of a 5% w/w solution prepared?**

   A A % w/w solution is defined as 1 g of solute per 100 g of solution (solute + solvent). A 5% w/w solution is prepared by weighing 5 g of the solute and adding it to 95 g of solvent (usually deionized water) to make a total solution weight of 100 g.

2. **Q** **How many grams of sodium chloride (NaCl) are needed to prepare 100 mL of a 0.9% w/v solution using deionized water as the solvent?**

A A % w/v solution is defined as 1 g of solute dissolved in 100 mL of solution. Therefore, 0.9 g of NaCl would be added and dissolved in a small amount of water in a 100 mL volummetric flask, and then additional water would be added to qs to the 100 mL mark on the flask.

3. **Q** **How many grams of potassium chloride (KCl) are present in 5 mL of a 25% w/v solution of KCl?**

A Since by definition a 25% w/v solution contains 25 g in 100 mL, by using ratio and proportion the amount of KCl present in 5 mL can be determined:

$$\frac{25.0 \text{ g}}{100 \text{ mL}} = \frac{X \text{ g}}{5 \text{ mL}}$$

By cross-multiplying, the following equation is derived:

$$(25)(5) = (100)(X)$$
$$125 = 100X$$
$$1.25 \text{ g} = X.$$

Therefore, there are 1.25 g of KCl in 5 mL of a 25% w/v solution.

4. **Q** **How is a 10% v/v solution of glacial acetic acid prepared using deionized water as the solvent?**

A By definition, a 10% v/v solution contains 1 mL of solute per 100 mL of solution. Therefore, a 10% v/v solution of glacial acetic acid contains 10 mL of glacial acetic acid added to 90 mL of water to make a total solution volume of 100 mL.

5. **Q** **How many milliliters of ethanol (EtOH) are needed to prepare a 70% v/v solution using deionized water as the diluent?**

A A 70% v/v solution of EtOH contains 70 mL of EtOH in 30 mL of water. Therefore, 70 mL of EtOH are necessary for this preparation.

6. **Q** **A total of 250 mL of a 35% v/v EtOH solution is needed. In the stockroom is a bottle of 70% v/v EtOH. How much of the 70% v/v EtOH should you use to prepare the 250 mL solution?**

A This problem is solved using a simple ratio and proportion calculation. The formula is:

$$C_1V_1 = C_2V_2$$

where:

C_1 = stock concentration
V_1 = volume of stock required

C_2 = concentration of the new solution

V_2 = volume of the new solution

By substituting into the equation the amounts given, the following equation is derived:

$$(70\%)(X) = (35\%)(250 \text{ mL})$$
$$(70)(X) = 8750$$
$$X = 125 \text{ mL.}$$

Therefore, 125 mL of the stock solution is added to a 250 mL volummetric flask. The remainder of the solution is deionized water (solvent), which is added until the 250 mL calibrated mark is reached.

7. **Q** **A total of 125 mL of a 10% solution is diluted to 500 mL in a 500 mL volummetric flask. What is the concentration of the new solution?**

A The formula $C_1V_1 = C_2V_2$ is used to solve this problem.

$$(10\% \text{ stock})(125 \text{ mL}) = (X)(500 \text{ mL})$$
$$1250 = (500)(X)$$
$$\frac{1250}{500} = 2.5.$$

Therefore, the new solution has a concentration of 2.5%.

PRACTICE PROBLEMS

Solve the following practice problems to further master the material. All answers and explanations to some problems can be found in a separate section at the back of the book.

1. How is a 15% w/w solution prepared?
2. How is a 15% w/v solution prepared?
3. How is a 15% v/v solution prepared?
4. How many milliliters of bleach are needed to prepare a 10% v/v solution using deionized water as the solvent?
5. Calculate the number of grams found in 100 mL of a 10% w/v solution of NaOH.
6. Calculate the number of grams found in 10 mL of a 20% w/v KCl solution.
7. Determine the amount of stock 80% v/v EtOH required to prepare 500 mL of a 20% v/v EtOH solution.
8. Determine the concentration of a diluted solution of Tris buffer if 300 mL of a 20% w/v Tris buffer solution is diluted to a final volume of 1000 mL.

Calculations Associated with Drug Dosages

CHAPTER 7

Interpreting Medical Orders

OBJECTIVES

Upon completion of this chapter, the reader should be able to:

1 Define common medical terms associated with prescriptions.

2 Describe the components of a prescription.

3 Translate verbal orders for drug dosages into practical applications by using ratio and proportion.

4 Translate orders from medical records into practical applications by using ratio and proportion.

INTRODUCTION

In a busy medical practice, clinic, or other health care setting, physicians may give medication orders, either verbally or in writing, that must be interpreted by other health care practitioners such as registered nurses, licensed practical nurses and medical assistants. All verbal orders are added to the patient's chart later on, becoming part of the permanent medical record. There are several things the health care practitioner must do to interpret the physician's order exactly. If it is a verbal order, the health care practitioner must understand both the name of the medication and the dose that has been prescribed. In addition, the frequency of the dose must be understood. Many medications are similar in name or appearance. Accurate verbal communication between the physician and the health care practitioner is vital to ensure that the correct medication is given. If the order is written, it will be found in the patient's chart. For an ambulatory outpatient, the order will be written by the physician as a prescription. Patients may question health care practitioners other than the prescribing physician about the order. It may be the responsibility of these individuals to educate the patient about how to take the medication.

Components of a Prescription

Figure 7-1 is a prescription for Tylenol 3, or Tylenol with codeine, a pain medication that is also a Drug Enforcement Agency (DEA) controlled substance. There are many different variations on a standard prescription, but they all have certain fixed elements. First is the name of the medical practice, the address, and the phone number. Next is the name of the physician, followed by the DEA number that allows the physician to write prescriptions for controlled substances. (If the prescription is for a medication that is not a controlled substance, the DEA number is not necessary.) In the body of the prescription, there is a space for the patient's name, address, and age (or birth date), as well as for the date the prescription is written. Below that is space for the prescription to be written and additional information including the number of refills. Finally, at the bottom, is an area for the physician's signature.

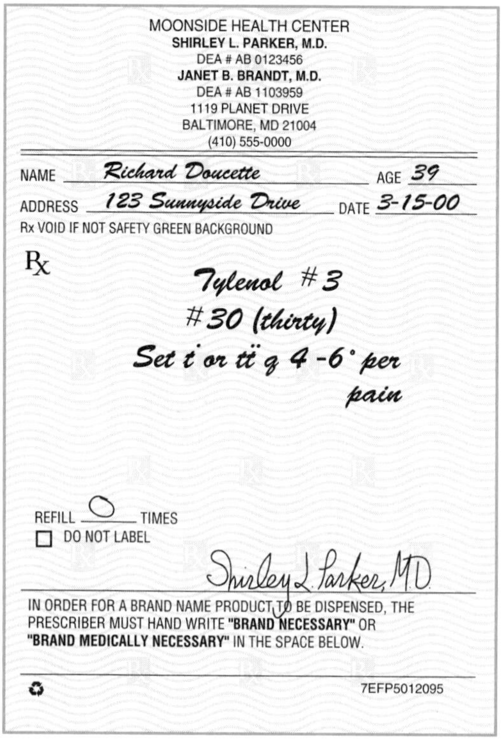
MOONSIDE HEALTH CENTER
SHIRLEY L. PARKER, M.D.
DEA # AB 0123456
JANET B. BRANDT, M.D.
DEA # AB 1103959
1119 PLANET DRIVE
BALTIMORE, MD 21004
(410) 555-0000

NAME *Richard Doucette* AGE *39*
ADDRESS *123 Sunnyside Drive* DATE *3-15-00*
Rx VOID IF NOT SAFETY GREEN BACKGROUND

℞
Tylenol #3
#30 (thirty)
Sig i or ii q 4-6° per pain

REFILL *0* TIMES
☐ DO NOT LABEL

Shirley L. Parker, MD

IN ORDER FOR A BRAND NAME PRODUCT TO BE DISPENSED, THE PRESCRIBER MUST HAND WRITE **"BRAND NECESSARY"** OR **"BRAND MEDICALLY NECESSARY"** IN THE SPACE BELOW.

7EFP5012095

FIGURE 7-1 Sample prescription.

Common Abbreviations Found in Prescriptions

Medicine has developed its own shorthand, both verbally and in writing, for frequently used terms or phrases. That is why it is very difficult for the average patient to read the prescription to be filled at the pharmacy and why the patient may ask for help in understanding how to take the medication at home. Health care practitioners must be able to interpret this shorthand accurately in order to educate the patient.

Medical shorthand is divided into two main categories: route of administration of the drug and frequency and/or timing of doses. Here are some of the most common abbreviations and their definitions.

ROUTE OF ADMINISTRATION

PO	=	by mouth
NPO	=	nothing by mouth
IV	=	by intravenous line
SL	=	sublingual, or under the tongue
SC	=	subcutaneous, or beneath the skin
IM	=	intramuscular, or into the muscle

FREQUENCY OR TIME OF DOSE

qam	=	take medication every morning
qpm	=	take medication every evening
ac	=	take medication before meals
pc	=	take medication after meals
prn	=	take medication as needed
hs	=	take medication before sleep
bid	=	take medication two times a day
tid	=	take medication three times a day
qid	=	take medication four times a day
qd	=	take medication every day
po	=	take medication by mouth

After a medication has been administered to a patient, it is recorded on the patient's chart. Figure 7-2 is an example of the charting of the administration of a medication order for 250 mg/mL of Mylanta antacid to be given po prn pc.

In most health care settings, stock quantities of medications are available so that the medical staff can dispense them to patients. The labels on medications have been standardized and contain important information. Figure 7-3 is a picture of a bottle of Biaxin.

Date	
2/15/00	250 mg/mL Mylanta po
	——————— S. Doucette, MA

FIGURE 7-2 Patient's medication order recorded on a patient chart.

Medication Labels

Each medication label contains the following information:

1. The generic name of the medication.
2. The trade name of the medication.
3. The name of the company that manufactured the medication.
4. The dosage of the medication.
5. The form (e.g., tablets, solution) in which the medication is dispensed.
6. The National Drug Code (NDC) number of medication.
7. The total quantity of medication, i.e., the number of tablets or milliliters in the medication bottle, vial, or ampule.

Sometimes the order calls for a medication dosage that is different from the stock dose. To conserve supplies, ratio and proportion calculations can be performed to use the available medications.

PROBLEMS

A nurse practitioner orders 500 mg acetaminophen for a patient to be taken prn for pain and asks the medical assistant to administer the first dose. The stock bottle contains acetaminophen tablets in a concentration of 250 mg. How many tablets does the medical assistant administer to the patient?

There are two ways to solve problems that involve dosage calculations. One is by the standard ratio and proportion method, as demonstrated in Chapters 3 and 6; the other is by using the following formula, as shown in Chapter 3:

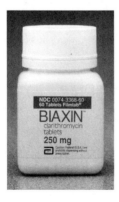

FIGURE 7-3 Biaxin drug label. (Courtesy of Abbott Laboratories, North Chicago, Illinois.)

$$\frac{\text{What you want}}{\text{What you have}} \times \underset{\text{(DF)}}{\text{Drug form}} = \underset{\text{(ADD)}}{\text{Amount of dispensed drug}}$$

> **Note** This formula should be used only when a single delivery method is being employed, such as tablets or capsules, at least until the student is very confident when using conversion math. Using this formula with more complex prescriptions, such as those for solutions of *X* g/L or *X* g per *Y* L, may be confusing, and it is recommended that straight ratio and proportion calculations be performed instead.

Using this formula to solve the medication problem results in the following equation:

$$\frac{500}{250} \times 1 \text{ tablet} = X \text{ ADD}$$

$$2 \text{ tablets} = \text{ADD}$$

Therefore, the nurse practitioner would dispense two 250 mg acetaminophen tablets to the patient.

By comparison, the use of the standard ratio and proportion calculation would result in the following equation:

$$\frac{250 \text{ mg}}{1 \text{ tablet}} = \frac{500 \text{ mg}}{X \text{ tablet(s)}}$$

Cross-multiplying the equations yields:

$$(250)X = 500(1)$$
$$X = \frac{500}{250}$$
$$= 2$$

Therefore, two 250 mg tablets are dispensed to yield a dosage of 500 mg.

An order is written for 1000 mg Depakote to be given to a patient. Figure 7-4 shows the stock bottle. How is this order dispensed?

Using the shortcut formula, the following equation is derived:

$$\frac{1000}{500} \times 1 \text{ tablet} = X \text{ ADD}$$

$$2 \text{ tablets} = \text{ADD}$$

Therefore, the patient would receive two 500 mg Depakote tablets for a dose of 1000 mg.

A physician assistant wants to administer a dose of 0.25 mg terbutaline IM to an asthmatic. On hand is a vial of terbutaline that contains 1 mg/mL. How does the physician assistant administer the 0.25 mg dose?

The ratio and proportion formula can be used to solve this problem. X is the amount of drug needed to dispense a 0.25 mg dose:

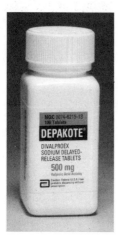

FIGURE 7-4 Depakote drug label. (Courtesy of Abbott Laboratories, North Chicago, Illinois.)

$$\frac{1\ mg}{1\ mL} = \frac{0.25\ mg}{X\ mL}$$

Cross-multiplying the equation yields:

$$(1)(X) = (1)(0.25)$$
$$X = 0.25\ mL$$

Therefore, the physician assistant administers 0.25 mL terbutaline IM to the patient.

A physician orders 20 mg furosimide (Lasix) IM for a patient. On hand is an ampule containing 4 mL with a concentration of 10 mg/mL. How does the medical assistant administer the dose?

$$\frac{10\ mg}{1\ mL} = \frac{20\ mg}{X\ mL}$$

Cross-multiplying the equation yields:

$$(10)(X) = (20)(1)$$
$$10X = 20$$
$$X = \frac{20}{10}$$
$$= 2$$

Therefore, the medical assistant administers 2 mL of the furosimide to the patient IM. This dose contains 20 mg of the medication.

Another question that can be asked is:

How much total drug is contained in the remaining 4 mL?

To determine this, first remember that the drug concentration is 10 mg/mL, i.e., for every 1 mL, there is 10 mg of drug in solution. Therefore, ratio and proportion can answer our question:

$$\frac{10\ mg}{1\ mL} = \frac{X\ mg}{4\ mL}$$

Cross-multiplying the equation yields:

$(1)(X) = (10)(4)$

$X = 40$

Therefore, a total of 40 mg of drug is contained in the remaining 4 mL of solution.

EXAMPLE PROBLEMS

This section is designed to be useful to both the student and the health care practitioner. Students can use the example problems in order to master the material. The health care practitioner can use these problems as templates for solving calculations. Find an example problem similar to the problem that you need to solve and substitute into the equation the numbers appropriate to your calculation.

1. **Q** **A physician orders amoxicillin 250 mg/dL tid. How often does the patient take the drug?**

   A TID means three times a day, or every 8 hours.

2. **Q** **A patient is NPO q12h prior to surgery. What does this mean?**

   A The patient should have nothing by mouth for 12 hours prior to surgery.

3. **Q** **A nurse practitioner prescribes 600 mg ibuprofen po q4h prn for a patient. The stock bottle contains ibuprofen tablets with a concentration of 300 mg. How many tablets does the nurse practitioner give the patient for the first dose?**

   A This problem can be solved by ratio and proportion or by the shortcut method derived from the ratio and proportion calculation. The shortcut formula is:

   $$\frac{\text{What you want}}{\text{What you have}} \times \text{Drug form} = \text{Amount of dispensed drug}$$
   $$(DF) \qquad\qquad (ADD)$$

   Substituting into the formula the values from the problem yields:

   $$\frac{600}{300} \times 1 \text{ tablet} = ADD$$

   2 tablets = amount to be dispensed.

   Therefore, two ibuprofen tablets are dispensed to the patient.

4. **Q** **A physician prescribes 800 mg Motrin for a patient. On hand is Motrin in 200 mg caplets. How is the dose dispensed to the patient?**

   A
   $$\frac{\text{Want}}{\text{Have}} \times 1 \text{ caplet} = X \text{ ADD}$$

   $$\frac{800 \text{ mg}}{200} \times 1 \text{ caplet} = X \text{ ADD}$$

   $$4 \text{ caplets} = X \text{ ADD}$$

Therefore the patient is given four 200 mg caplets for a total 800 mg dose of Motrin.

5. **Q** **A physician orders Bromfed-DMB cough syrup to be given to a 22-year-old woman at a dosage and rate of 10 mg/mL po q4h. The stock Bromfed-DMBO contains 5 mg/mL. How is the medication dispensed?**

A Ratio and proportion can be used to solve this problem.

$$\frac{5 \text{ mg}}{1 \text{ mL}} = \frac{10 \text{ mg}}{X \text{ mL}}$$

Cross-multiplying the equation yields:

$$5(X) = 10$$

$$X = \frac{10}{5}$$

$$= 2.$$

Therefore, the patient would receive 2 mL of the medication q4h.

PRACTICE PROBLEMS

Solve the following problems to further master the material. All answers and explanations to some problems can be found in a separate section at the back of the book.

Define the following abbreviations.

1. tid
2. SL
3. bid
4. prn
5. po
6. q4h

Given the following situations, how would you dispense the ordered medication?

7. Ordered 250 mg caplets; on hand are 125 mg caplets.
8. Ordered 500 mg tablets; on hand are 1000 mg tablets scored in half.
9. Ordered 100 mg tablets; on hand are 25 mg tablets.
10. Ordered 10 mg liquid cough medicine; on hand is 20 mg/mL cough medicine.

CHAPTER **8**

Medication Preparation and Routes of Administration

INTRODUCTION

Millions of medications are dispensed every day to patients around the world. These medications are in three basic forms: liquid, as in oral medications or intravenous (IV) fluids; solids, as in tablets, capsules, or caplets; and semisolid form, as in ointments or suppositories. Physicians and others who are legally able to prescribe medication for patients write orders for dosages of these drugs that may not be the same as the dosage of the medication that is available. Therefore, sometimes mathematical conversions must be performed to dispense the dosage of the drug that was ordered. Sometimes the pharmacist prepares the dosage and performs these calculations, but it is important that all health care practitioners who administer or oversee the administration of medications thoroughly understand the conversion process.

Calculating Oral Dosages

Solid Medication

Oral dosages are dosages of medication that are taken by mouth. Solid medications, as noted above, can take the form of a tablet, capsule, or caplet. The route of administration may be either sublingual, as with nitroglycerin, or oral. Children's medications in tablet form are frequently designed to be chewed and then swallowed, while medications designed for adults are typically swallowed whole.

Some tablets are *scored*, i.e., marked by lines to allow them to be cut in half or in fourths. If a tablet is scored in half, the dosage will be cut in half if a patient takes only half of the tablet. Never cut unscored tablets, as these tablets are designed to be taken whole.

PROBLEMS

An order is written for 325 mg acetaminophen q4h. On hand are 650 mg acetaminophen tablets. How is the medication administered?

Acetaminophen tablets are scored to allow administration of half of the stated dose. Using ratio and proportion, the following equation is derived:

$$\frac{650 \text{ mg}}{1 \text{ tablet}} = \frac{325 \text{ mg}}{X \text{ tablet}}$$

Cross-multiplying the equation yields:

$$(650)(X) = (325)(1)$$
$$650X = 325$$
$$X = \frac{325}{650}$$
$$= 1/2$$

Therefore, the 650 mg tablet would be scored in half to dispense a 325 mg dose.

This same problem can be solved using the shortcut formula:

$$\frac{\text{What you want}}{\text{What you have}} \times \text{Drug form} = \text{Amount of dispensed drug}$$
$$\text{(DF)} \qquad \text{(ADD)}$$

Using this formula, the following equation is derived:

$$\frac{325}{650} \times 1 \text{ tablet} = X \text{ ADD}$$
$$1/2 \text{ tablet} = X \text{ ADD}$$

Therefore, one-half of a 650 mg tablet is dispensed to yield a 325 mg dose.

A patient has been prescribed rifabutin in a dosage of 300 mg qd. The medication is available in 150 mg capsules. How is the drug administered?

Using the shortcut formula:

$$\frac{300 \text{ mg}}{150 \text{ mg}} \times \text{capsules} = X \text{ ADD}$$

$$X = 2 \text{ capsules}$$

Therefore, the patient would take two capsules of rifabutin each day to reach the prescribed dose.

A patient recently diagnosed with epilepsy is placed on phenytoin to be administered by 50 mg chewable tablets, not to exceed a maximum dosage of 600 mg daily. How many tablets can the patient take without exceeding the maximum dosage?

Ratio and proportion can be used to solve this problem.

$$\frac{50 \text{ mg}}{1 \text{ tablet}} = \frac{600 \text{ mg}}{X \text{ tablets}}$$

Cross-multiplying the equation yields:

$$(50)(X) = (1)(600)$$
$$50X = 600$$
$$X = \frac{600}{50}$$
$$= 12$$

The patient can safely chew up to 12 tablets per day without exceeding the maximum dosage.

A 55-year-old man is prescribed valproic acid at a dosage of 15 mg/kg body mass/day. The patient weighs 74 kg. How many milligrams of valproic acid per day should this patient receive?

Ratio and proportion can be used to solve this problem.

$$\frac{15 \text{ mg}}{1 \text{ kg}} = \frac{X \text{ mg}}{74 \text{ kg}}$$

Cross-multiplying the equation yields:

$$X = (15)(74)$$
$$= 1110$$

Therefore, the patient receives 1110 mg of valproic acid per day.

Liquid Medication

Liquid medication is medication that is dissolved in a solvent. The solvent may be water or alcohol based. Liquid medications may be dispensed either orally, via injection, or via intravenous lines. The dosages of many liquid medications are calculated on the basis of the patient's weight in kilograms to ensure that a sufficient quantity of the medication is present in the body.

Prescriptions for oral medications may be written to be dispensed in either metric or nonmetric units. However, most patients are not familiar with the metric system and may need help in understanding exactly how much of the medication to take. The following box lists common units ordered for oral medications, and Table 8-1 is a conversion chart between the two systems.

> **COMMON UNITS FOR ORAL MEDICATIONS**
>
> Drop (gtt)
> Teaspoon (tsp)
> Tablespoon (tbsp)
> Ounce (oz)
> Milligram (mg)
> Gram (g)

PROBLEMS

A patient infected with the human immunodeficiency virus (HIV) is prescribed the antiviral medication Norvir (see Figure 8-1). The bottle of Norvir contains 80 mg/ mL, and the prescribed dosage is 800 mg po tid. How is this medication dispensed?

First, determine exactly what the prescription calls for. In this case, it is for 800 mg given by mouth three times a day, or every 8 hours.

Next, determine how to dispense this medication using the information provided on the medication label. The medication is in a solution of 80 mg/mL. Therefore, using

TABLE 8-1   Conversion Chart between Common Units for Oral Medications

Unit	Equivalent Unit
60 drops	1 teaspoon
3 teaspoons	1 tablespoon
2 tablespoons	1 ounce
5 mL	1 teaspoon
15 mL	1 tablespoon
30 mL	1 ounce

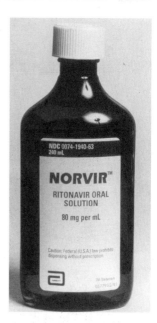

FIGURE 8-1 Norvir drug label. (Courtesy of Abbott Laboratories, North Chicago, Illinois.)

ratio and proportion, the number of milliliters needed for an 800 mg dose can be determined:

$$\frac{80 \text{ mg}}{1 \text{ mL}} = \frac{800 \text{ mg}}{X \text{ mL}}$$

Cross-multiplying the equation yields:

$$(80)(X) = (1)(800)$$
$$80X = 800$$
$$X = \frac{800}{80}$$
$$= 10$$

Therefore, the patient must take 10 mL of Norvir every 8 hours. But how should this medication be taken? Table 8-1 shows that 1 teaspoon is equal to 5 mL. Since the patient must take 10 mL of this liquid suspension three times a day, a dosage schedule of 2 teaspoons (10 mL) three times a day would fulfill the dosage requirement.

A 16-year-old girl is prescribed amoxicillin for an ear infection at a dosage of 500 mg po tid. The liquid elixir contains amoxicillin at a concentration of 250 mg/5 mL. How is the prescribed dosage administered?

Using ratio and proportion, the following equation is derived:

$$\frac{250}{5 \text{ mL}} = \frac{500}{X \text{ mL}}$$

Cross-multiplying the equation yields:

$$(250)(X) = (500)(5)$$
$$250X = 2500$$
$$X = 10$$

Therefore, 10 mL, or 2 teaspoons of amoxicillin, are administered every 8 hours.

Calculating Parenteral Dosages of Medications

Parenteral medications are administered by routes other than the oral/gastrointestinal route. They are usually administered by intramuscular (IM), subcutaneous (SC), or intradermal injection. They can also be administered through a continuous intravenous (IV) line. Vaccinations, allergy tests, and tuberculin skin tests are a few of the situations involving parenteral medications. The medication may come in prepackaged syringes, ampules, or vials containing the powdered medication, which must be reconstituted with diluent prior to use (see Figure 8-2).

Syringes for administration of parenteral medication range from 1 cc tuberculin or insulin syringes to 3 cc, 5 cc, and 10 cc syringes. One cc syringes are marked in 0.01 cc increments, while the other syringes are marked in 0.1 cc increments (see Figure 8-3).

Dosages for parenteral medications are calculated both for volume of liquid injected and for quantity by weight of the dissolved medication. For example, medication A may be given at a dosage of 2.5 mg/mL, while medication B may be dispensed at a dosage of 0.1 g/mL. As mentioned previously, some medications are also prescribed as dosage/body weight. For example, an antihistamine may be administered as X mg/kg.

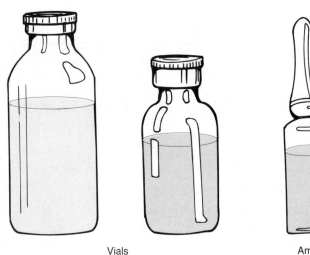

Vials   Ampule

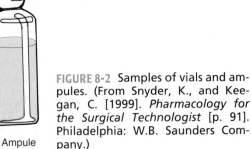

FIGURE 8-2 Samples of vials and ampules. (From Snyder, K., and Keegan, C. [1999]. *Pharmacology for the Surgical Technologist* [p. 91]. Philadelphia: W.B. Saunders Company.)

A. Insulin

B. Tuberculin

C. 3cc Luerlock

D. 10cc Plain tip

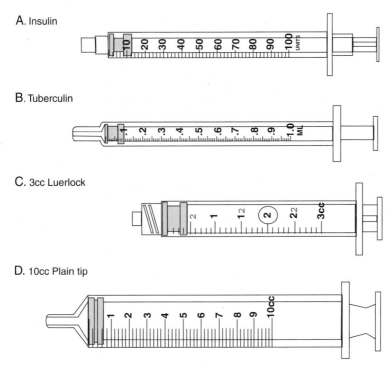

FIGURE 8-3 Samples of syringes. (From Snyder, K., and Keegan, C. [1999]. *Pharmacology for the Surgical Technologist* [p. 98]. Philadelphia: W.B. Saunders Company.)

PROBLEMS

A 10-year-old boy is brought into the emergency room in an acute asthmatic crisis. The physician orders a 5 mg/kg loading dose of theophylline via IV line. The boy weighs 80 pounds. How much theophylline is administered?

In order to calculate the dosage, the weight in pounds must be converted into kilograms. The conversion chart (Table 4-3) in Chapter 4 lists the conversion factor from pounds to kilograms as 0.453. Therefore, multiply the number of pounds by 0.453 to calculate the weight in kilograms.

$$80 \text{ lb} \times 0.453 = 36.24 \text{ kg, or rounded to } 36 \text{ kg}$$

Ratio and proportion can also be used to convert pounds to kilograms:

$$\frac{2.2 \text{ lb}}{1 \text{ kg}} = \frac{80 \text{ lb}}{X \text{ kg}}$$

$$2.2X = (80)(1)$$

$$X = \frac{80}{2.2}$$

$$= 36$$

Next, use ratio and proportion to determine the dosage:

$$\frac{5 \text{ mg}}{1 \text{ kg}} = \frac{X \text{ mg}}{36 \text{ kg}}$$

Cross-multiplying the equation yields:

$$X = (5)(36)$$
$$= 180$$

Therefore, the boy is given 180 mg theophylline.

Furosemide at a dosage of 40 mgq12h IM has been ordered for a 50-year-old woman. The medication is available in vials containing 10 mg/mL. How is this medication administered?

Using ratio and proportion:

$$\frac{10 \text{ mg}}{1 \text{ mL}} = \frac{40 \text{ mg}}{X \text{ mL}}$$

Cross-multiplying the equation yields:

$$(10)(X) = (40)(1)$$
$$10X = 40$$
$$X = \frac{40}{10}$$
$$= 4$$

Therefore, 4 mL furosemide is administered IM to this woman every 12 hours.

A patient is prescribed valproic acid at a dose of 15 mg/kg/day. The patient weighs 85 kg. How much valproic acid is administered per day?

Using ratio and proportion:

$$\frac{15 \text{ mg}}{1 \text{ kg}} = \frac{X \text{ mg}}{85 \text{ kg}}$$

Cross-multiplying the equation yields:

$$X = (15)(85)$$
$$= 1275$$

Therefore, 1275 mg or 1.275 g of valproic acid is administered per day.

A diabetic is told to use 40 units of insulin. The only syringe he has on hand is not an insulin syringe but a 1 cc syringe. Can he still use this syringe, and if so, how many cubic centimeters of insulin should he administer?

Insulin typically is formulated in 100 unit dosages, with specialized syringes calibrated to deliver 100 units marked in 10 unit intervals. The conversion between units and milliliters (or cubic centimeters, an older but comparable term) is:

100 units = 1 mL

Therefore, it is acceptable, but not usual, to use a 1 cc syringe to administer insulin. To calculate the dosage, use ratio and proportion:

$$\frac{100 \text{ units}}{1 \text{ mL}} = \frac{40 \text{ units}}{X \text{ mL}}$$

Cross-multiplying the equation yields:

$$(100)(X) = (40)(1)$$
$$100X = 40$$
$$X = \frac{40}{100}$$
$$= 0.4$$

Therefore, 40 units of insulin is equal to 0.4 mL of insulin.

Maintaining Intravenous Lines

Medications or fluids given via IV lines need to be carefully calculated to prevent over- or underdosing the patient. In previous years, if patients required IV lines, they were usually hospitalized; in today's health care environment, they may be just as likely to receive IV therapy at home. In the past, IV fluid entered the patient's body through the use of gravity. The IV bag was placed on a pole higher than the patient's body, the IV needle was inserted into a vein, and the fluid was allowed to flow into the vein. The rate at which the fluid flowed into the vein was controlled by a valve system at a flow rate of X drops per minute. The drops per minute (gtt/min) were calculated by the following formula:

$$\text{Drops/min} = \frac{\text{IV infused (mL)} \times \text{gtt/mL}}{\text{Total time for infusion in minutes (or no. of hours} \times 60 \text{ min/hr})}$$

For example, if 150 mL of D_5W is to be infused in 1 hour with a drop factor of 10 gtt/mL, then the number of drops administered per minute would be:

$$\text{Drops/min} = \frac{150 \text{ mL} \times 10 \text{ gtt/mL}}{60 \text{ min}}$$
$$= \frac{1500}{60}$$
$$= 25$$

Therefore, the flow rate would be 25 gtt/min.

The health care practitioner would have to monitor the gravity-fed IV setup continuously to ensure that it was running properly. The gravity method has been replaced in many settings by an IV pump. The pump infuses the IV fluid at a rate that is set by the operator and needs less oversight than the gravity method.

PROBLEMS

What would the flow rate be for 200 mL D₅W at 15 gtt/mL over 1 hour?

Using the formula, the following equation is derived:

$$\text{Drops/min} = \frac{200 \text{ mL} \times 15 \text{ gtt/mL}}{60 \text{ min}}$$

$$= \frac{3000}{60}$$

$$= 50 \text{ gtt/min}$$

Therefore, the IV would be set to dispense 50 drops/min for 1 hour. Standard IV tubing dispenses 10, 15, or 20 drops/mL. A microdrip IV apparatus is available if less than 50 mL of fluid per hour is to be infused and dispenses at a rate of 60 drops/mL.

How many drops per minute will it take to dispense 30 mL of fluid using a micro-drip IV tubing set at 60 gtt/mL for 1 hour?

The same formula can be used to solve this equation:

$$\text{Drops/min} = \frac{30 \text{ mL} \times 60 \text{ gtt/mL}}{60 \text{ min}}$$

$$= \frac{1800}{60}$$

$$= 30$$

Therefore, the IV would be set to dispense 30 drops/min.

How many mL/hr would be infused in a patient receiving 10,000 units of heparin in 500 mL D₅W at a rate of 0.20 unit/kg/min? The patient weighs 80 kg, and the IV is being infused at a rate of 60 gtt/min.

To solve this equation, first determine the total concentration per minute.

$$\frac{0.20 \text{ units/min}}{1 \text{ kg}} = \frac{X \text{ units/min}}{80}$$

Cross-multiplying the equation yields:

$$(1)(X) = (0.20)(80)$$
$$X = 16$$

Therefore, the concentration of heparin is 16 units/min. Therefore, the total amount of heparin infused per hour is 16 units/min × 60 minutes = 960 units/hr.

Next, determine the concentration of heparin per milliliter. If 10,000 units of heparin are contained in 500 mL, then:

$$\frac{10,000 \text{ units}}{500 \text{ mL}} = \frac{X}{1 \text{ mL}}$$

Cross-multiplying the equation yields:

$$(500)(X) = (10,000)(1)$$

$$X = \frac{10,000}{500}$$

$$= 20 \text{ units/mL}$$

Therefore, the heparin is being infused at a concentration of 20 units/mL.

Finally, determine the amount in milliliters of heparin infused per hour. Twenty units/mL are being infused with a total concentration of 960 units/hr. Therefore:

$$\frac{20 \text{ units}}{1 \text{ mL}} = \frac{960 \text{ units}}{X \text{ mL}}$$

$$(20)X = 960$$

$$X = \frac{960}{20}$$

$$= 48$$

Therefore, the heparin is being infused at a rate of 48 mL/hr.

Calculating Pediatric Dosages

Some medications can be administered to both adults and children. However, the dosage must be changed because of children's smaller height and lower weight. Otherwise, children may be accidentally overmedicated. Figure 8-4 is a nomogram that can be used to correct for children's smaller body surface area.

To use the nomogram, the child's height in centimeters or inches is required, as well as the weight in kilograms or pounds. Find the child's height and weight on the nomogram. Using a ruler as a straight edge, line up the height and weight on the ruler. The surface area is the third scale, or the center scale for children of normal height and weight, and the child's body surface area is found at the intersection of the scale and the ruler.

PROBLEM

A 4-year-old boy with acute lymphoblastic leukemia (ALL) is being treated with methotrexate. The standard dose is 3.3 mg/m². The child weighs 24 kg and is 33 inches tall. How much methotrexate should be administered?

Using the nomogram, the body surface area is determined to be 0.8. Therefore, the calculation to determine the medication dosage is:

$$\frac{3.3 \text{ mg}}{1 \text{ m}^2} = \frac{X \text{ mg}}{0.8 \text{ m}^2}$$

Cross-multiplying the equation yields:

$$X = (3.30)(0.8)$$

$$= 2.64 \text{ mg}$$

Therefore, the child would receive 2.64 mg of methotrexate.

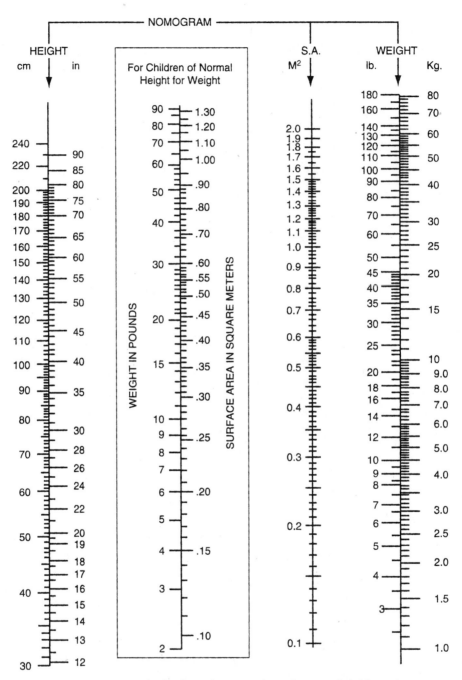

FIGURE 8-4 Nomogram for body surface area for infants and children. (From Kee, J. L., and Marshall, S. M. [1996]. *Clinical Calculations: With Applications to General and Specialty Areas* [3rd ed., p. 198]. Philadelphia: W.B. Saunders Company.)

EXAMPLE PROBLEMS

This section is designed to be useful to both the student and the health care practitioner. Students can use the example problems in order to master the material. The health care practitioner can use these problems as templates for solving calculations. Find an example problem similar to the problem that you need to solve and substitute into the equation the numbers appropriate to your calculation.

1. **Q** **An order is written for 500 mg aspirin po tid. On hand are 1000 mg tablets that are scored. How is this medicine administered?**

   A Ratio and proportion can be used to solve this problem.

   $$\frac{500 \text{ mg}}{1 \text{ tablet}} = \frac{1000 \text{ mg}}{X \text{ tablet}}$$

   Cross-multiplying the equation yields:

   $$(500)(X) = 1000$$
   $$X = \frac{1000}{500}$$
   $$= \frac{1}{2}$$

   The 1000 mg tablet is cut in half to administer a 500 mg dose.

2. **Q** **An order is written to administer 250 mg Tylenol po tid. On hand are 125 mg Tylenol caplets. How is the Tylenol administered?**

   A This problem can be solved using either ratio and proportion or the shortcut formula:

   $$\frac{\text{What you want}}{\text{What you have}} \times \underset{\text{(DF)}}{\text{Drug form}} = \underset{\text{(ADD)}}{\text{Amount of dispensed drug}}$$

   Substituting into the formula yields the following equation:

   $$\frac{250 \text{ mg}}{125 \text{ mg}} \times 1 \text{ caplet} = \text{ADD}$$
   $$2 \text{ caplets} = \text{ADD}.$$

3. **Q** **A patient has been prescribed a drug for pain management that has a maximum safe daily dosage of 1500 mg. The patient can take the medication prn but cannot exceed the safe dose. The medication is available in 250 mg scored tablets. How many tablets can the patient safely take each day?**

   A The shortcut formula can be used to solve this problem.

   $$\frac{1500 \text{ mg}}{250 \text{ mg}} \times 1 \text{ tablet} = \text{ADD}$$
   $$6 \text{ tablets} = \text{ADD}.$$

   Therefore, the patient can take no more than six tablets a day.

4. **Q** An order is written to administer 10 mg diazepam IM to a 55-year-old man to relieve his acute anxiety concerning a scheduled sigmoidoscopy. On hand is a vial of diazepam with a concentration of 5 mg/mL. How many milliliters of diazepam are injected?

A Ratio and proportion can be used to solve this problem.

$$\frac{5 \text{ mg}}{1 \text{ mL}} = \frac{10 \text{ mg}}{X \text{ mL}}$$

Cross-multiplying the equation yields:

$$(5)(X) = (10)(1)$$

$$X = \frac{10}{5}$$

$$= 2 \text{ mL.}$$

Therefore, 2 mL of diazepam would be injected IM.

5. **Q** An order is written for 25 mg haloperidol IM qd for a patient in a psychiatric ward. On hand is a vial of haloperidol with a strength of 50 mg/mL. How is the ordered dose of haloperidol administered?

A Using ratio and proportion:

$$\frac{50 \text{ mg}}{1 \text{ mL}} = \frac{25 \text{ mg}}{X \text{ mL}}$$

Cross-multiplying the equation yields:

$$(50)(X) = (25)(1)$$

$$X = \frac{25}{50}$$

$$= 0.5.$$

Therefore, 0.5 mL of 50 mg/mL haloperidol is administered to deliver the ordered dose.

6. **Q** A physician assistant diagnoses a young child with acute otitis media. He writes a prescription to treat the infection with erythromycin at a dosage of 50 mg/kg in three divided doses tid for 10 days. The child weighs 30 kg. If the oral suspension for erythromycin is available at a concentration of 250 mg/5 mL, how should the pharmacist fill the prescription?

A First, the pharmacist would calculate the total dosage. Since the order is for 50 mg/kg, ratio and proportion would be used to calculate the total dosage:

$$\frac{50 \text{ mg}}{1 \text{ kg}} = \frac{X}{30 \text{ kg}}$$

Cross-multiplying the equation yields:

$$(X)(1) = (50)(30)$$
$$X = 1500.$$

Therefore, a total quantity of 1500 mg/day is ordered.

Next, the pharmacist needs to fill the order with the available medication of 250 mg/5 mL erythromycin. Ratio and proportion can be used to determine the actual dosage given tid.

$$\frac{250 \text{ mg}}{5 \text{ mL}} = \frac{1500 \text{ mg}}{X \text{ mL}}$$

Cross-multiplying the equation yields:

$$(250)(X) = (1500)(5)$$
$$250X = 7500$$
$$X = 30 \text{ mL per day, or 300 mL for a 10-day dose.}$$

Since the total dose is to be divided into three doses per day, 10 mL of erythromycin is to be given to the child three times a day.

7. **Q** **What is the formula used to calculate the flow rate of IV fluids?**

   A The formula to calculate the flow rate of IV fluids is:

   $$\text{Drops/min} = \frac{\text{IV infused (mL)} \times \text{drops/mL (gtt/mL)}}{\text{Total time for infusion in minutes}}$$

8. **Q** **A patient is to be given an IV of 500 mL D$_5$W at 20 gtt/mL over 8 hours. What is the flow rate?**

   A Using the formula yields:

   $$\text{Drops/min} = \frac{500 \text{ mL} \times 20 \text{ gtt/mL}}{480 \text{ min}}$$
   $$= \frac{10,000}{480}$$
   $$= 20.8 \text{ or } 21 \text{ gtt/min.}$$

9. **Q** **1 g lidocaine in 250 mL D$_5$W with a flow rate of 5 mg/min is to be infused. How many milligrams will be infused per hour?**

   A Since 5 mg is infused per minute, 5 × 60 minutes = 300 mg is infused per hour.

10. **Q** **Using the information given in question 9, how many milliliters per hour will be infused?**

    A We know that 300 mg of lidocaine is infused per hour. However, we want the volume in milliliters infused per hour. First, we must calculate the concentration of lidocaine in milligrams per milliliter. We know that there are 1000 mg of lidocaine in 250 mL D$_5$W. Therefore, to find out how many milligrams there are in 1 mL of lidocaine we use ratio and proportion:

$$\frac{1000 \text{ mg}}{250 \text{ mL}} = \frac{X}{1 \text{ mL}}$$

Cross-multiplying the equation yields:

$$(250)(X) = (1000)(1)$$
$$X = \frac{1000}{250}$$
$$= 4.$$

Therefore, there are 4 mg/mL of lidocaine in this IV.

Last, determine the number of milliliters of lidocaine infused per hour. We know that there are 4 mg/mL and that they are infused at a rate of 300 mg/hr. Therefore, divide the number of milligrams per hour by the concentration to determine the number of milliliters per hour:

$$\frac{300 \text{ mg/hr}}{4 \text{ mg/mL}} = 75 \text{ mL/hr}.$$

Therefore, the IV is infused at a rate of 75 mL/hr.

11. **Q** **A child with a weight of 40 kg and a height of 45 inches is given a standard dose of 2.5 mg/m² of a chemotherapy drug. How much of the drug would be administered?**

   A Using the nomogram (Figure 8-4), the child's surface area is found to be 1.2 m². Therefore, the calculation to determine the medication dosage is:

$$\frac{2.5 \text{ mg}}{1 \text{ m}^2} = \frac{X \text{ mg}}{1.2 \text{ m}^2}$$

Cross-multiplying the equation yields:

$$(1)(X) = (2.5)(1.2)$$
$$X = 3 \text{ mg}.$$

Therefore, the child would receive 3 mg of the chemotherapy drug.

PRACTICE PROBLEMS

Solve the following problems to further master the material. All answers and explanations to some problems can be found in a separate section at the back of the book.

Given the following situations, how would you dispense the ordered medication?

1. Ordered 500 mg tablets; on hand are 1000 mg tablets to be given q4h.
2. Ordered 0.25 mg of drug A qd; on hand is 0.125 mg drug A in tablet form.

3. Ordered 30 mg/kg/day of drug Y. The patient weighs 110 pounds.
4. Ordered 1 g/kg/day of drug B. The patient weighs 22 kg.
5. How many milliliters are in a teaspoon?
6. How many milliliters are in a tablespoon?
7. If an elixir has a concentration of 25 mg/mL and the dosage is 500 mg qid, how is the medication administered?
8. An order is written for 10 mg/kg of drug C for a patient who weighs 75 kg. How is the medication administered?
9. A patient is prescribed WonderDrug at a dose of 40 mg/kg/day. The patient weighs 165 pounds. How is the medication administered?
10. Calculate the flow rate per minute in an IV of 150 mL normal saline at a rate of 20 gtt/mL over 1 hour.
11. Calculate the rate in mL/hr of an IV containing 5 mg/mL of drug D in 500 mL of D_5W at a rate of 0.5 mg/min.
12. A child weighing 15 kg and 28 inches tall must receive 2.5 mg/m^2 of a chemotherapy drug. How is the drug administered?

Laboratory Calculations

CHAPTER **9**

Clinical Chemistry Laboratory

OBJECTIVES

Upon completion of this chapter, the reader should be able to:

1 Calculate the anion gap of unknown samples.

2 Calculate serum osmolality concentrations.

3 Calculate the osmolal gap in patient samples.

4 Calculate the concentration of LDL and VLDL cholesterol.

ANION GAP

CALCULATED OSMOLALITY AND OSMOLAL GAP

Calculated Osmolality
Osmolal Gap

LIPID CALCULATIONS

EXAMPLE PROBLEMS

PRACTICE PROBLEMS

REFERENCES

BIBLIOGRAPHY

INTRODUCTION

The field of clinical chemistry includes a large variety of test methods. A detailed discussion of topics such as spectrophotometry, enzyme kinetics, and acid-base balance is beyond the scope of this chapter. Today, most clinical chemistry tests are performed on automated instruments, and while an understanding of these topics is helpful to the health care worker who is performing laboratory tests using automated instruments, it is not necessary. Instead, all health care workers who perform laboratory tests must be trained to use maintenance and trouble-shooting procedures on the many instruments whose peak performance is essential to ensure accurate, precise laboratory results. However, if a laboratory method is not automated and is performed manually, a complete understanding of the theory behind the analysis will enhance the accuracy and precision of the assay. This chapter will concentrate on those clinical chemistry calculations that may be performed manually, either as quality assurance mechanisms, to assist the physician in providing a correct diagnosis, or as a means of producing a laboratory result. Additional information on calculations performed in the clinical chemistry laboratory can be found in many clinical chemistry textbooks, as well as in the textbook *Mathematics for the Clinical Laboratory* published in 1997 by W.B. Saunders Company.

Anion Gap

Many functions of the human body are regulated by systems that work to maintain a neutral environment. For example, plasma glucose is regulated by two pancreatic peptides: insulin, which decreases the plasma glucose level, and glucagon, which increases the plasma glucose level. The body also tries to maintain electrolyte neutrality. The concentration of anions (negatively charged molecules) should equal the concentration of cations (positively charged molecules) in the body.

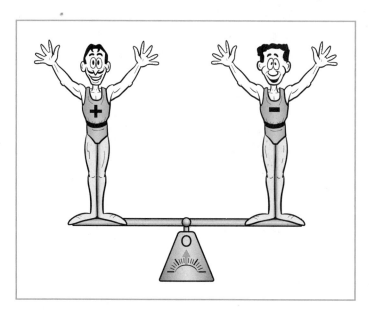

This balance is measured by the *anion gap*. The anion gap does not measure all anions or cations in the body, but just those that have the highest concentration and the potential to alter the balance significantly. The most abundant cation in the blood is sodium (Na^+); the most abundant anion is chloride (Cl^-). Bicarbonate (HCO_3^-), another anion, is also included in the anion gap. Some laboratories include potassium (K^+) in the anion gap. However, the concentration of potassium is relatively low compared to that of the other electrolytes. The anion gap is calculated as follows:

$$[Na^+] - ([Cl^-] + [HCO_3^-]) = \text{anion gap}$$

or

$$([Na^+] + [K^+]) - ([Cl^-] + [HCO_3^-]) = \text{anion gap}$$

The reference range for the anion gap calculated without potassium is 8–16 mmol/L, and the reference range for the anion gap calculated with potassium is 10–20 mmol/L.[1] The anion gap is useful to detect changes in the concentration of unmeasured anions and cations. For example, an elevated anion gap is due to the presence of other anions, such as proteins or, most commonly, acids such as ketoacids. A decreased anion gap may be due to an increase in unmeasured cations such as magnesium or calcium. In addition, the anion gap may be used as a quality assurance measure to ensure the reliability of the electrodes that determine electrolyte concentration.

PROBLEMS

Calculate the anion gap for a 58-year-old insulin-dependent diabetic woman who is admitted to the emergency room in a comatose state.

Her electrolyte profile is:

Sodium = 135 mmol/L
Potassium = 3.5 mmol/L
Chloride = 102 mmol/L
Bicarbonate = 15 mmol/L

To compare formulas, the anion gap will be calculated using both formulas.

Calculated Anion Gap without Potassium

Anion gap = 135 − (102 + 15)
= 135 − 117
= 18 mmol/L (reference range: 8–16 mmol/L)

Calculated Anion Gap with Potassium

Anion gap = (135 + 3.5) − (102 + 15)
= 138.5 − 117
= 21.5 mmol/L (reference range: 10–20 mmol/L)

Calculate the anion gap for a John Doe admitted to the trauma center following a serious automobile accident.

Sodium = 147 mmol/L
Potassium = 5.5 mmol/L
Chloride = 110 mmol/L
Bicarbonate = 14 mmol/L

Both formulas will be used to demonstrate the calculation of the anion gap. However, remember that in the laboratory, the anion gap will be calculated using one formula or the other, but not both.

Anion Gap without Potassium

$$\text{Anion gap} = 147 - (110 + 14)$$
$$= 147 - 124$$
$$= 23 \text{ mmol/L (reference range: 8–16 mmol/L)}$$

Calculated Anion Gap with Potassium

$$\text{Anion gap} = (147 + 5.5) - (110 + 14)$$
$$= 152.5 - 124$$
$$= 28.5 \text{ mmol/L (reference range: 10–20 mmol/L)}$$

Calculated Osmolality and Osmolal Gap

Calculated Osmolality

The osmolality of a solution is based on the number of dissolved particles in a solution, not on the size, weight, or ionic activity of the particles. The unit of measurement is the osmol. Osmolality measures the *total* concentration of all of the ions and molecules present in serum or urine. Some substances, like glucose, do not dissociate, or split apart in solution, so each particle of glucose is equal to 1 osmolal. Other substances, such as sodium chloride, dissociate into a sodium particle and a chloride particle, so one particle of sodium chloride would equal a 2 osmolal solution. Sodium, glucose, and urea are major contributors to the total osmolality of serum. Because the major contributors to serum osmolality are tightly regulated, the osmolality of serum can be calculated.

$$\text{Osmolality (mOsmol/kg } H_2O) = 1.86\,[Na^+] + \frac{[\text{glucose}]}{18} + \frac{[\text{BUN}]}{2.8}$$

The factor 1.86 is used because each sodium ion is balanced by an anion, but dissociation is not perfect. The factor 18 is used because the molecular weight of glucose is approximately 180 and the factor of 18 converts mg/dL, the unit used for glucose measurements, to mmol/L, the unit used for osmolality measurements. The molecular weight of blood urea nitrogen (BUN) is approximately 28; thus 2.8 is used.

This formula cannot be used for calculating urine osmolality because the concentration of particles varies greatly, depending on the patient's hydration status.

PROBLEMS

A 78-year-old man was admitted to the emergency room suffering from heat stroke. Based on the patient's laboratory results, what is the patient's serum osmolality?

The laboratory results were as follows:

Sodium = 162 mEq/L
Potassium = 5.8 mEq/L
Glucose = 110 mg/dL
BUN = 16 mg/dL

To calculate the serum osmolality, use the following formula and substitute into it the data from the problem:

$$\text{Osmolality (mOsmol/kg } H_2O) = 1.86 \, [Na^+] + \frac{[\text{glucose}]}{18} + \frac{[\text{BUN}]}{2.8}$$

$$= (1.86)(162) + \frac{110}{18} + \frac{16}{2.8}$$

$$= 301 + 6.1 + 5.8$$

Calculated serum osmolality = 313 mOsmol/kg H_2O

(reference range for patients > 60 = 280–301 mOsm/kg)[2]

The calculated osmolality is elevated above the reference range and reflects the patient's dehydrated status.

A 36-year-old insulin-dependent diabetic was brought to the emergency room in a diabetic coma. Based on the patient's laboratory values, what is the patient's serum osmolality?

The laboratory results were as follows:

Sodium = 145 mEq/L
Potassium = 4.5 mEq/L
Glucose = 750 mg/dL
BUN = 25 mg/dL

To calculate the serum osmolality, use the following formula and substitute into it the data from the problem:

$$\text{Osmolality (mOsmol/kg } H_2O) = 1.86 \, [Na^+] + \frac{[\text{glucose}]}{18} + \frac{[\text{BUN}]}{2.8}$$

$$= (1.86)(145) + \frac{750}{18} + \frac{25}{2.8}$$

$$= 270 + 41.7 + 8.9$$

$$= 321 \text{ mOsmol/kg } H_2O$$

(reference range for adults = 275–295 mOsm/kg)

This patient's abnormally elevated glucose concentration caused the serum osmolality to be elevated as well.

Osmolal Gap

The *osmolal gap* is the difference between the calculated osmolality and the measured osmolality. The average osmolal gap is 0–10 mOsm/kg H_2O. Elevation of the gap is usually due to factors other than sodium, glucose, or BUN. The presence of ketones or alcohols such as ethanol (EtOH) in the serum can elevate the osmolal gap. The osmolal gap may also be useful as a quality assurance measure to detect technical errors.

PROBLEMS

 A 35-year-old woman was found unconscious and admitted to the hospital. Based on her laboratory results, what is the patient's osmolal gap?

The patient's laboratory results were as follows:

$$\begin{aligned}
\text{Sodium} &= 142 \text{ mEq/L} \\
\text{Potassium} &= 4.5 \text{ mEq/L} \\
\text{Glucose} &= 105 \text{ mg/dL} \\
\text{BUN} &= 12 \text{ mg/dL} \\
\text{Serum osmolality} &= 320 \text{ mOsm/kg} \\
\text{Serum EtOH} &= 160 \text{ mg/dL}
\end{aligned}$$

To calculate the osmolal gap, first calculate the osmolality:

$$\text{Osmolality (mOsmol/kg } H_2O) = 1.86 \, [Na^+] + \frac{[\text{glucose}]}{18} + \frac{[\text{BUN}]}{2.8}$$

$$= (1.86)(142) + \frac{105}{18} + \frac{12}{2.8}$$

$$= 264 + 5.8 + 4.3$$

$$= 274 \text{ mOsm/kg}$$

$$\text{Osmolal gap} = \text{calculated osmolality} - \text{measured osmolality}$$

$$= 320 - 274 \text{ mOsm/kg}$$

$$= 46 \text{ mOsm/kg}$$

The osmolal gap, 46 mOsm/kg, indicates the presence of other dissolved particles in the serum. The elevated EtOH concentration is probably the cause of the increased osmolal gap.

An 18-month-old boy was rushed to the emergency room because of suspected poisoning due to ingestion of antifreeze after his father found him unconscious in the family's garage. What is the patient's osmolal gap?

The patient's laboratory results were as follows:

$$\begin{aligned}
\text{Sodium} &= 138 \text{ mEq/L} \\
\text{Potassium} &= 3.9 \text{ mEq/L} \\
\text{Glucose} &= 115 \text{ mg/dL} \\
\text{BUN} &= 10 \text{ mg/dL} \\
\text{Serum osmolality} &= 260 \text{ mOsm/kg}
\end{aligned}$$

To calculate the osmolal gap, first calculate the osmolality:

$$\text{Osmolality (mOsmol/kg H}_2\text{O)} = 1.86\,[\text{Na}^+] + \frac{[\text{glucose}]}{18} + \frac{[\text{BUN}]}{2.8}$$

$$= (1.86)(138) + \frac{115}{18} + \frac{10}{2.8}$$

$$= 257 + 6.4 + 3.6$$

$$= 267 \text{ mOsm/kg}$$

$$\text{Osmolal gap} = \text{Calculated osmolality} - \text{measured osmolality}$$

$$= 260 - 267 \text{ mOsm/kg}$$

$$= 7 \text{ mOsm/kg}$$

A positive or negative sign is associated with the osmolal gap. Therefore, the gap, 7 mOsm/kg, does not have a negative sign in front of it even though, mathematically, it could.

This osmolal gap falls within the normal range for the osmolal gap. Therefore, it is highly unlikely that the toddler was poisoned by ingesting the antifreeze.

Lipid Calculations

Coronary artery disease (CAD) is one of the leading causes of death today. Consequently, patients and their doctors are very interested in laboratory tests that can detect risk factors for CAD. Total cholesterol, high density lipoprotein (HDL) cholesterol, low density lipoprotein (LDL) cholesterol, and triglycerides are commonly measured to determine this risk. Currently, only a few methods are available to directly measure LDL cholesterol. Instead, LDL cholesterol is calculated by the Friedewald[3] formula.

$$\text{LDL cholesterol} = \text{total cholesterol} - \left(\text{HDL} + \frac{\text{triglycerides}}{5}\right)$$

The triglycerides/5 fraction is an estimation of very low density lipoprotein (VLDL) cholesterol. This formula is not accurate if the triglyceride level is above 300 mg/dL and assumes that no other source of triglycerides, such as chylomicrons, are present. Since chylomicrons are the major transporters of dietary fat and are rich in exogenous triglycerides (i.e., those outside the body), patients must fast to eliminate the presence of chylomicrons.

PROBLEMS

A 43-year-old man with a family history of CAD. Calculate the patient's LDL cholesterol level.

The patient's lipid profile analysis is as follows:

Total cholesterol = 345 mg/dL
Triglycerides = 230 mg/dL
HDL cholesterol = 70 mg/dL

To do this, use the previously given formula:

$$\text{LDL cholesterol} = \text{Total cholesterol} - \left(\text{HDL} + \frac{\text{Triglycerides}}{5}\right)$$

$$= 345 \text{ mg/dL} - (70 \text{ mg/dL} + 230 \text{ mg/dL} \div 5)$$
$$= 345 \text{ mg/dL} - (70 \text{ mg/dL} + 46 \text{ mg/dL})$$
$$= 345 \text{ mg/dL} - 116 \text{ mg/dL}$$
$$= 229 \text{ mg/dL}$$

Calculate the LDL cholesterol level of a 52-year-old woman taking estrogen replacement therapy.

The patient has the following lipid profile:

Total cholesterol = 225 mg/dL
Triglycerides = 180 mg/dL
HDL cholesterol = 54 mg/dL

To do this, use the previously given formula:

$$\text{LDL cholesterol} = \text{Total cholesterol} - \left(\text{HDL} + \frac{\text{Triglycerides}}{5}\right)$$

$$= 225 \text{ mg/dL} - (54 \text{ mg/dL} + 180 \text{ mg/dL} \div 5)$$
$$= 225 \text{ mg/dL} - (54 \text{ mg/dL} + 36 \text{ mg/dL})$$
$$= 225 \text{ mg/dL} - 90 \text{ mg/dL}$$
$$= 135 \text{ mg/dL}$$

The National Cholesterol Education Program has established the acceptable ranges for triglycerides and cholesterol to reduce the incidence of CAD.[4] A total cholesterol value below 200 mg/dL is desirable, values between 200 and 240 mg/dL indicate a borderline high risk, and those above 240 mg/dL place the patient at high risk of developing CAD. In addition, an LDL cholesterol value below 130 mg/dL is desirable, values between 130 and 150 mg/dL are borderline high risk, and those above 150 mg/dL place the patient at high risk for developing CAD. The patient discussed above has both elevated total cholesterol and elevated LDL cholesterol, which places her at high risk of developing CAD.

EXAMPLE PROBLEMS

This section is designed to be useful to both the student and the health care practitioner. Students can use the example problems in order to master the material. The health care practitioner can use these problems as templates for solving calculations. Find an example problem similar to the problem that you need to solve and substitute into the equation the numbers appropriate to your calculation.

1. **Q** **What is the anion gap of a sample with $[Na^+]$ = 141 mmol/L, $[Cl^-]$ = 101 mmol/L, and $[HCO_3^-]$ = 25 mmol/L?**

   A The anion gap is a useful calculation for detecting changes in the concentration of unmeasured anions and cations. In the body, the concentration of cations should equal that of anions. In some disease states and medical conditions, this balance may be altered. For example, in ketoacidosis, there is an increase in the concentration of ketoacids in the blood. These anions are not normally measured, so the anion gap will be increased. Using the data from the problem, the calculated anion gap is:

   $$\text{Anion gap} = 141 \text{ mmol/L} - (101 + 25 \text{ mmol/L})$$
   $$= 141 - 126$$
   $$= 15 \text{ mmol/L.}$$

2. **Q** **Two anion gap calculations are currently in use. One uses the potassium value and the other does not. Using the same anion and cation values in example problem 1, calculate the anion gap using the formula that includes potassium, given the potassium value of 4.5 mmol/L.**

   A The anion gap calculation that includes potassium is:

   $$([\text{Sodium}] + [\text{Potassium}]) - ([\text{Chloride}] + [HCO_3^-]) = \text{Anion gap}$$

   Substituting the values from the previous question, the anion gap can be calculated:

   $$\text{Anion gap} = (141 + 4.5 \text{ mmol/L}) - (101 + 25 \text{ mmol/L})$$
   $$= 145.5 - 126$$
   $$= 19.5 \text{ mmol/L.}$$

3. **Q** **Calculate the anion gap using the formula without potassium for the following values:**

   $$Na = 152 \text{ mmol/L}$$
   $$K = 4.1 \text{ mmol/L}$$
   $$Cl = 112 \text{ mmol/L}$$
   $$HCO_3^- = 28 \text{ mmol/L}$$

   A The anion gap is calculated as follows:

   $$\text{Anion gap} = 152 \text{ mmol/L} - (112 + 28 \text{ mmol/L})$$
   $$= 152 - 140$$
   $$= 12 \text{ mmol/L.}$$

4. **Q** **Using the laboratory values from example problem 3, calculate the anion gap using the formula that includes potassium.**

   A   Anion gap = (152 + 4.1 mmol/L) − (112 + 28 mmol/L)

   $$= 156.1 - 140$$

   $$= 16 \text{ mmol/L}.$$

5. **Q** **Calculate the osmolal gap of a patient with measured serum osmolality of 294 mOsm/kg, Na^+ of 157 mmol/L, K^+ of 6.8 mmol/L, glucose of 132 mg/dL, and BUN of 14.2 mg/dL.**

   A   The osmolal gap is the difference between the calculated osmolality and the measured osmolality. The reference range for the osmolal gap is −10 to +10 mOsmol/kg H_2O. Theoretically, there should be no difference between the measured and calculated serum osmolalities. The constituents of the calculation comprise the majority of dissolved solutes in the blood. When other nonmeasured solutes are present, such as EtOH, the measured serum osmolality value will differ from the calculated osmolality value. The formula used to calculate osmolality is:

   $$\text{Osmolality} = 1.86 \, [Na^+] + \frac{[\text{glucose}]}{18} + \frac{[\text{BUN}]}{2.8}$$

   Substituting into the formula the values from the problem yields the following equation:

   $$\text{Osmolality} = (1.86)(157 \text{ mmol/L}) + \frac{132 \text{ mg/dL}}{18} + \frac{14.2 \text{ mg/dL}}{2.8}$$

   $$= 292 + 7.3 + 5.1$$

   $$= 304 \text{ mOsm/kg } H_2O.$$

   Next, the osmolal gap is calculated by determining the difference between the calculated osmolality and the measured osmolality.

   $$\text{Osmolal gap} = \underset{\text{(calculated)}}{304 \text{ mOsm/kg } H_2O} - \underset{\text{(measured)}}{294 \text{ mOsm/kg } H_2O}$$

   $$= 10 \text{ mOsm/kg } H_2O.$$

6. **Q** **Calculate the osmolal gap of a patient with measured serum osmolality of 345 mOsm/kg, Na^+ of 134 mmol/L, K^+ of 3.5 mmol/L, glucose of 473 mg/dL, and BUN of 11.5 mg/dL.**

   A   First, calculate the serum osmolality using the osmolality formula and the patient's values.

   $$\text{Osmolality} = (1.86) \, (134 \text{ mmol/L}) + \frac{473 \text{ mg/dL}}{18} + \frac{11.5 \text{ mg/dL}}{2.8}$$

   $$= 249.2 + 26.3 + 4.1$$

   $$= 280 \text{ mOsm/kg } H_2O.$$

Next, subtract the calculated osmolality from the measured osmolality to determine the osmolal gap.

$$\text{Osmolal gap} = \underset{\text{(calculated)}}{345 \text{ mOsm/kg H}_2\text{O}} - \underset{\text{(measured)}}{280 \text{ mOsm/kg H}_2\text{O}}$$

$$= 65 \text{ mOsm/kg H}_2\text{O}.$$

7. Q **What is the concentration of LDL cholesterol in a sample whose total cholesterol is 225 mg/dL, HDL cholesterol is 40 mg/dL and triglyceride concentration is 175 mg/dL?**

A Currently, there are only a few direct LDL cholesterol assays. Instead, the LDL cholesterol concentration is determined mathematically using the triglyceride concentration. To determine the accurate triglyceride concentration, i.e., one in which dietary triglycerides do not interfere, a fasting specimen is required. Therefore, a fasting specimen is also required for an accurate LDL cholesterol calculation. The formula used to determine the LDL cholesterol concentration is:

$$\text{LDL cholesterol} = \text{Total cholesterol} - \left(\text{HDL} + \frac{\text{Triglycerides}}{5}\right)$$

The Triglycerides/5 fraction represents the VLDL fraction of cholesterol. This measure is valid only if the triglyceride concentration is below 400 mg/dL. Therefore, the patient's LDL cholesterol is:

$$\text{LDL cholesterol} = 225 \text{ mg/dL} - \left(40 \text{ mg/dL} + \frac{175 \text{ mg/dL}}{5}\right)$$

$$= 225 - (40 + 35)$$
$$= 225 - 75$$
$$= 150 \text{ mg/dL.}$$

8. Q **What is the concentration of LDL cholesterol in a sample whose total cholesterol is 160 mg/dL, HDL cholesterol is 25 mg/dL, and triglyceride concentration is 125 mg/dL?**

A $\text{LDL cholesterol} = 160 \text{ mg/dL} - \left(25 \text{ mg/dL} + \frac{125 \text{ mg/dL}}{5}\right)$

$$= 160 - (25 + 25)$$
$$= 160 - 50$$
$$= 110 \text{ mg/dL.}$$

Solve the following problems to further master the material. All answers and explanations to some problems can be found in a separate section at the back of the book.

Calculate the anion gap for each of the following groups of laboratory values, first using the formula without potassium and then using the formula that includes potassium:

1. Na^+ = 152 mmol/L, K^+ = 4.2 mmol/L, Cl^- = 105 mmol/L, HCO_3^- = 34 mmol/L.
2. Na^+ = 132 mmol/L, K^+ = 3.4 mmol/L, Cl^- = 101 mmol/L, HCO_3^- = 28 mmol/L.
3. Na^+ = 145 mmol/L, K^+ = 4.0 mmol/L, Cl^- = 110 mmol/L, HCO_3^- = 36 mmol/L.
4. Na^+ = 160 mmol/L, K^+ = 6.7 mmol/L, Cl^- = 108 mmol/L, HCO_3^- = 31 mmol/L.

Calculate the serum osmolality of the following groups of laboratory data:

5. Na^+ = 147 mmol/L, glucose = 110 mg/dL, BUN = 15 mg/dL.
6. Na^+ = 137 mmol/L, glucose = 148 mg/dL, BUN = 21 mg/dL.
7. Na^+ = 145 mmol/L, glucose = 472 mg/dL, BUN = 25 mg/dL.
8. Na^+ = 165 mmol/L, glucose = 80 mg/dL, BUN = 11 mg/dL.

Calculate the osmolal gap of the following groups of laboratory data:

9. Na^+ = 149 mmol/L, glucose = 115 mg/dL, BUN = 10 mg/dL, and measured osmolality = 290 mOsm/kg.
10. Na^+ = 152 mmol/L, glucose = 106 mg/dL, BUN = 15 mg/dL, and measured osmolality = 310 mOsm/kg.
11. Na^+ = 151 mmol/L, glucose = 163 mg/dL, BUN = 18 mg/dL, and measured osmolality = 285 mOsm/kg.
12. Na^+ = 135 mmol/L, glucose = 95 mg/dL, BUN = 18 mg/dL, and measured osmolality = 265 mOsm/kg.

Calculate the LDL cholesterol concentration of the following groups of laboratory data:

13. Total cholesterol = 195 mg/dL, HDL cholesterol = 45 mg/dL, and triglycerides = 150 mg/dL.
14. Total cholesterol = 248 mg/dL, HDL cholesterol = 52 mg/dL, and triglycerides = 265 mg/dL.
15. Total cholesterol = 160 mg/dL, HDL cholesterol = 55 mg/dL, and triglycerides = 110 mg/dL.

16. Total cholesterol = 360 mg/dL, HDL cholesterol = 72 mg/dL, and triglycerides = 380 mg/dL.

REFERENCES

1. C. A. Burtis and E. R. Ashwood. *Tietz Textbook of Clinical Chemistry*, 3rd ed. W.B. Saunders Company, Philadelphia, 1999.
2. Ibid.
3. W. T. Friedewald, R. I. Levy, and D. S. Frederickson. Estimation of the concentration of low-density lipoprotein cholesterol in plasma without use of the preparative ultracentrifuge. *Clin Chem* 18:499, 1972.
4. Report of the National Cholesterol Treatment Program Expert Panel on Detection, Evaluation, and Treatment of High Blood Cholesterol in Adults. *Arch Intern Med* 148:36–39, 1988.

BIBLIOGRAPHY

Anderson, S., and Cockayne, S. *Clinical Chemistry: Concepts and Applications*. W.B. Saunders Company, Philadelphia, 1993.

Henry, J. *Clinical Diagnosis and Management by Laboratory Methods*, 19th ed. W.B. Saunders Company, Philadelphia, 1996.

Kaplan, L., and Pesce, A. *Clinical Chemistry: Theory, Analysis and Correlation*, 3rd ed. C.V. Mosby Company, St. Louis, 1996.

CHAPTER **10**

Urinalysis Laboratory

OBJECTIVES

Upon completion of this chapter, the reader should be able to:

1 Define the following terms: clearance, glomerular filtration rate, intrinsic clearance, extrinsic clearance.

2 State the clearance formula.

3 Calculate uncorrected creatinine clearance rates.

4 Utilize a nomogram to calculate corrected creatinine clearance rates.

5 Correct urinometer readings due to temperature variations and increased glucose and protein concentrations.

URINE TESTS

Quantitative Chemical Analyses
Calculating the Quantity per Volume of
 Collected Urine Analytes
Calculating the Quantity of Urine Collected per
 Unit of Collection Time
Converting the Quantity of Analyte Measured
 in mg/dL into g/Day

RENAL FUNCTION TESTS

**CORRECTIONS USED FOR THE REFRACTOMETER
AND URINOMETER**

Calibration
Correction for Temperature
Correction for Protein
Correction for Glucose

EXAMPLE PROBLEMS

PRACTICE PROBLEMS

BIBLIOGRAPHY

INTRODUCTION

Urine Tests

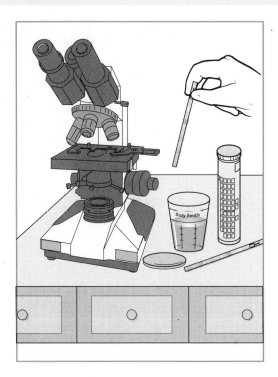

Urinalysis is one of the most common laboratory tests performed. Chemically impregnated strips allow the laboratorian to screen the urine for chemical constituents. Microscopic evaluation of sediment aids in determining the cellular constituents of the urine. Routine urinalysis is an excellent screening tool for many different diseases and conditions such as diabetes, urinary tract infections, metabolic disorders, and liver disorders. However, for patients who have renal disease, more definitive tests must be performed.

Quantitative Chemical Analyses

The physician may request a quantitative analysis of a constituent found in urine. For example, a 24 hour sample collected for total protein analysis or for urea may be ordered. The urine sample is analyzed for the particular constituent, but additional mathematical calculations must be performed before the result is recorded. Because the volume and collection period of the urine sample are variable, the test result must be standardized to allow comparison of results. Most urine test results are recorded as quantity of analyte per unit of time, usually 24 hours or 1 day. Occasionally, a urine sample will be collected for a shorter time period. In that case, the test result can be reported as the quantity per volume of collection or as the quantity per unit of time.

Calculating the Quantity per Volume of Collected Urine Analytes

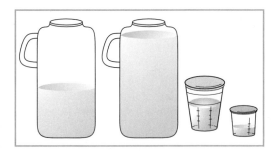

In general, if a nonelectrolyte is measured in urine, it is reported in units of mg/day or in the international units of mmol/day. Urine electrolytes are generally reported in units of mEq/day or mmol/day. If urine is not collected for a full 24 hour collection, the results may be extrapolated for a 24 hour collection for compounds that are excreted uniformly during this period and reported in terms of volume collected or quantity per total time collected. To calculate the quantity per volume collected, a ratio and proportion calculation can be performed.

PROBLEMS

A urine specimen collected over 12 hours with a volume of 525 mL is analyzed for creatinine. The result is 65 mg/dL. What is the result in terms of milligrams per volume of collection?

To solve this problem, a ratio and proportion calculation is performed. Remember, units must be the same; therefore, convert deciliters into milliliters (1 dL = 100 mL).

$$\frac{65 \text{ mg}}{100 \text{ mL}} = \frac{X \text{ mg}}{525 \text{ mL}}$$

Cross-multiplying the equation yields:

$$(65)(525) = (100)(X)$$
$$34125 = (100)(X)$$
$$341 = X$$

Therefore, there are 341 mg of creatinine per 525 mL of urine.

A urine specimen collected over 12 hours with a volume of 735 mL is analyzed for total protein. The result is 25 mg/L. What is the result in terms of milligrams per volume of collection?

As shown in the problem above, a ratio and proportion calculation is performed. Remember, units must be the same; therefore, convert liters into milliliters (1 L = 1000 mL).

$$\frac{25\ mg}{1000\ mL} = \frac{X\ mg}{735\ mL}$$

Cross-multiplying the equation yields:

$$(25)(735) = (1000)(X)$$
$$18375 = (1000)(X)$$
$$18 = X$$

Therefore, there are 18 mg of protein per 735 mL of urine.

Calculating the Quantity of Urine Collected per Unit of Collection Time

This calculation is identical to the previous calculation except that instead of being reported as milligrams per volume of collection, the result is reported as milligrams per collection time.

As calculated in the first example, a urine specimen collected over 12 hours with a volume of 525 mL has a creatinine concentration of 65 mg/dL, or 341 mg/525 mL. Since the 525 mL was collected over 12 hours, the result can also be recorded as 341 mg/12 hours.

As calculated in the second example, a urine specimen collected over 12 hours with a volume of 735 mL has a total protein concentration of 25 mg/L, or 18 mg/735 mL. Since the 735 mL was collected over 12 hours, the result can also be recorded as 18 mg/12 hours.

Converting the Quantity of Analyte Measured in mg/dL into g/Day

The quantity of an analyte measured in mg/dL can be converted into g/day by using the following conversion formula:

$$\frac{X\ analyte\ mg}{dL} \times \frac{mL\ collected}{24\ hour\ collection\ time} \times \frac{1\ dL}{100\ mL} \times \frac{g}{1000\ mg} = g/day$$

PROBLEMS

A urine urea value of 800 mg/dL is obtained from a urine sample with a volume of 1200 mL collected for 24 hours. What is the urine urea value in g/day?

Substituting into the conversion formula, the following formula is derived:

$$\frac{800 \text{ mg}}{\text{dL}} \times \frac{1200 \text{ mL}}{24 \text{ hr}} \times \frac{1 \text{ dL}}{100 \text{ mL}} \times \frac{1 \text{ g}}{1000 \text{ mg}}$$

$$= \frac{(800 \text{ g})(1200)(1)}{100{,}000}$$

$$= 9.6 \text{ g/24 hr}$$

Therefore, the urine urea concentration is 9.6 g/day or 9.6 g per 24 hours of collection.

A urine uric acid value of 90 mg/dL is obtained from a urine specimen with a volume of 1750 mL collected for 24 hours. What is the urine uric acid value in g/day?

Substituting into the conversion formula, the following formula is derived:

$$\frac{90 \text{ mg}}{\text{dL}} \times \frac{1750 \text{ mL}}{24 \text{ hr}} \times \frac{1 \text{ dL}}{100 \text{ mL}} \times \frac{1 \text{ g}}{1000 \text{ mg}}$$

$$= \frac{(90 \text{ g})(1750)(1)}{100{,}000}$$

$$= 1.5 \text{ g/24 hr}$$

Therefore, the urine uric acid concentration is 1.5 g/day or 1.5 g/24 hours of collection.

Renal Function Tests

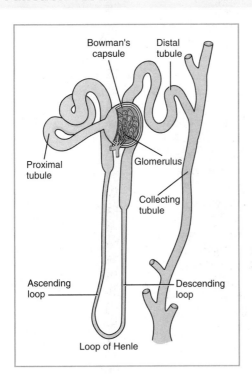

One of the most common renal function tests is the *clearance test*. This test provides information on the glomerular and tubular function of the kidneys. The kidney tubules' main function is to excrete waste products while reabsorbing water and dissolved chemicals from the ultrafiltrate. By measuring the concentration per unit of time in urine of a chemical that will be removed, or "cleared," by the kidney tubules, the physiologic function of the tubules can be determined.

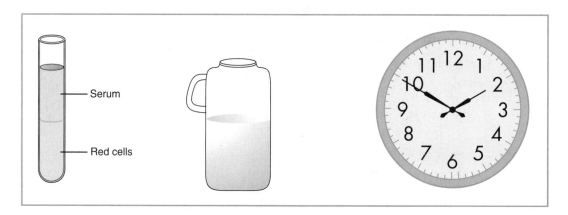

There are many variations on the clearance test. All of them measure three parameters: the plasma (or serum) concentration of the chemical to be cleared, the urine concentration of that chemical, and the clearance time. In this manner, the *glomerular filtration rate (GFR)* can be determined. This is the rate at which chemicals are filtered or "cleared" from the kidney. The clearance tests differ from one another in terms of the chemical to be cleared by the kidney and analyzed. Chemicals that are foreign to the body and completely cleared are measured by *extrinsic clearance tests*. These chemicals include inulin and *p*-aminohippurate. The chemical is injected into the patient intravenously, and its concentration in plasma is measured. All urine is collected during the clearance procedure, and the volume is measured. After the time interval, which may be 6, 12, or 24 hours, the urine and plasma are analyzed for the chemical concentration. *Intrinsic clearance tests* measure chemicals that are intrinsic to the body, such as creatinine and urea. The urea clearance test was one of the first clearance tests performed. Since approximately 40% of urea is reabsorbed into the renal tubules, urea clearance tests do not provide a full assessment of clearance. Creatinine is a waste product of muscle metabolism. It is produced at a constant rate and in proportion to muscle mass. Very little creatinine is secreted by the tubular cells; therefore, the concentration of creatinine in urine provides an excellent assessment of the tubular excretion function and the GFR. As in extrinsic clearance tests, the plasma levels of creatinine or urea are determined. Urine is collected for a fixed time period of 6, 12, or 24 hours. The 24 hour period is the most common time interval. The urine concentration of urea or creatinine is also determined.

All clearances are calculated by the following formula:

$$\frac{UV}{P}$$

Where:

U = urine concentration in mg/dL of the analyte cleared
V = volume of urine in mL/min
P = plasma concentration of the analyte in mg/dL

PROBLEMS

A urine specimen for a creatinine clearance test was collected over 24 hours. The total volume of urine is 2100 mL. The plasma creatinine concentration is 1.8 mg/dL, and the urine creatinine concentration is 155 mg/dL. What is the creatinine clearance?

To solve this problem, first determine the volume of urine per mL/min. Divide 2100 by 1440 to obtain the volume in mL/min because in 24 hours there are 1440 minutes (24 × 60).

$$mL/min = \frac{2100}{1440} = 1.46 \text{ mL/min}$$

Next, use the formula to obtain the creatinine clearance value.

$$\frac{UV}{P} = \frac{(155 \text{ mg/dL}) \ 1.46 \text{ mL/min}}{1.8 \text{ mg/dL}} = 125.7 \text{ mL/min}$$

Therefore, the creatinine clearance is 126 mL/min.

A urine specimen for a creatinine clearance test was collected over 12 hours. The total volume of urine is 0.430 L, the plasma creatinine concentration is 4.1 mg/dL, and the urine creatinine concentration is 130 mg/dL. What is the creatinine clearance rate?

To solve this problem, first determine the volume of urine per mL/min. In 12 hours there are 720 minutes (60 minutes × 12 hours). Divide 430 mL by 720 to determine the amount of urine produced in mL/min.

$$\frac{430}{720} = 0.60 \text{ mL/min (volume of urine)}$$

Using the clearance formula and substituting in the numbers:

$$\text{Clearance (mL/min)} = \frac{130 \text{ mg/dL} \times 0.60 \text{ mL/min}}{4.1 \text{ mg/dL}}$$

$$= 19.0 \text{ mL/min}$$

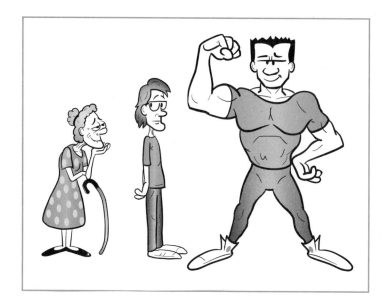

This formula was developed for use in patients with an adult average body size of 1.73 square meters (m²). Patients with a larger than average or smaller than average body size would have inaccurate clearance values if this formula is used alone. In addition, this formula cannot be used to determine the clearance values of children due to their much smaller body size. Figure 10-1 is a nomogram that can be used to compensate for body sizes different from 1.73 m². To use the nomogram, the patient's height in centimeters or inches is required, as well as his or her weight in kilograms or pounds. Find the patient's height and weight on the nomogram. Using a ruler as a straight edge, line up the height and weight on the ruler. The surface area is the center scale, and the patient's body surface area is found at the intersection of the scale and the ruler.

PROBLEMS

A creatinine clearance test was ordered for an obese kidney patient. Her weight was 350 pounds, and her height was 5 feet 6 inches. Her 24 hour urine volume was 1650 mL, plasma creatinine concentration was 7.8 mg/dL, and urine creatinine concentration was 120 mg/dL. What is this patient's creatinine clearance rate?

To solve this problem, first determine the volume of urine creatinine in mL/min.

$$\text{Urine creatinine} = \frac{1650 \text{ mL}}{(60)(24)} = \frac{1650}{1440} = 1.15 \text{ mL/min}$$

Next, use Figure 10-1 to determine the patient's body surface area. The nomogram consists of three scales. The first one, on the left side of the nomogram, is the height scale. Height can be measured in feet and inches as well as in centimeters. The scale on the right side of the nomogram is the weight scale. Weight can be

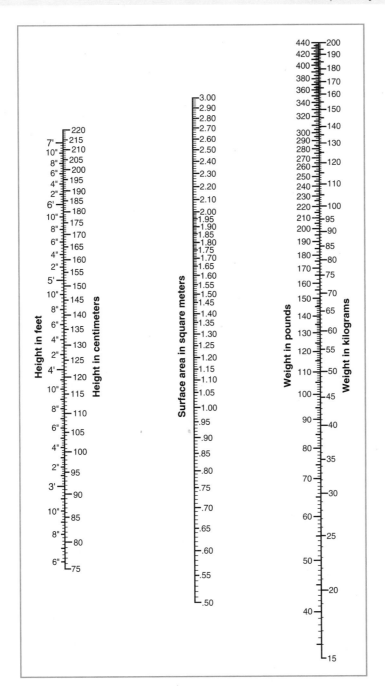

FIGURE 10-1 Nomogram for the determination of body surface areas. (From Doucette, L. J. [1997]. *Mathematics for the Clinical Laboratory* [p. 186]. Philadelphia: W.B. Saunders.)

measured both in pounds and in kilograms. The middle scale is the body surface area scale. To determine the patient's body surface area, first find the patient's height in feet and inches on the scale to the left. Next, find the patient's weight on the scale to the right. Then, using a straight edge, draw a line through the body surface area scale connecting both measurements. The point of intersection through the body surface area scale will be the patient's body surface area. This patient has a body surface area of 2.34 m². Finally, use the corrected clearance formula to determine the clearance rate.

$$\text{Corrected creatinine clearance} = \frac{UV}{P} \times \frac{1.73 \text{ m}^2}{2.34 \text{ m}^2}$$

Using the values given, the formula becomes:

$$\frac{(120 \text{ mg/dL})(1.15 \text{ mL/min})}{7.8} \times \frac{1.73 \text{ m}^2}{2.34 \text{ m}^2}$$

$$= 17.7 \text{ mL/min} \times 0.739$$

$$= 13.1 \text{ mL/min corrected creatinine clearance}$$

Note that the corrected clearance value is lower than the uncorrected value because of the patient's increased body size.

A creatinine clearance test is ordered for an elderly female patient who is 5 feet tall and weighs 87 pounds. Her urine creatinine concentration is 170 mg/dL, plasma creatinine concentration is 1.3 mg/dL, and urine volume on a 12 hour collection is 515 mL. What is her corrected creatinine clearance rate?

To solve this problem, first determine the quantity of urine per minute.

$$\text{Urine/min} = \frac{515}{(60)(12)} = 0.72 \text{ mL/min}$$

Because this patient does not have an average body size, a corrected version of the clearance formula will be used to obtain her creatinine clearance rate. Often, the height and weight of patients are not known to the laboratory. Clearances are then reported as uncorrected for body size. To correct for body size, use Figure 10-1 to determine the corrected body size. By drawing a line between the patient's height and weight, it can be determined that this patient has a body surface area of 1.25 m². Next, use the modified creatinine clearance formula:

$$\frac{UV}{P} \times \frac{1.7 \text{ m}^2}{1.25 \text{ m}^2} = \frac{(170 \text{ mg/dL})(0.72 \text{ mL/min})}{1.3 \text{ mg/dL}} \times 1.36$$

$$= \frac{122 \text{ mL/min}}{1.3} \times 1.36$$

$$= 128.0 \text{ mL/min corrected creatinine clearance}$$

What is this patient's uncorrected clearance rate?

To determine the uncorrected clearance rate, do not correct for body surface area. Use the unmodified clearance formula. Without the correction factor for her smaller than average body surface area of 1.36 m², this patient's uncorrected clearance rate is 94.2 mL/min.

Corrections Used for the Refractometer and Urinometer

Calibration

When urinalysis is performed, the specific gravity of the urine is measured. The specific gravity is important because it indicates the quantity of dissolved solids in the urine such as urea and chloride. A urinometer can be used to measure the specific gravity of urine. This instrument consists of a small cylindrical tube in which the urine is placed and a modified hydrometer float (see Figure 10-2). This

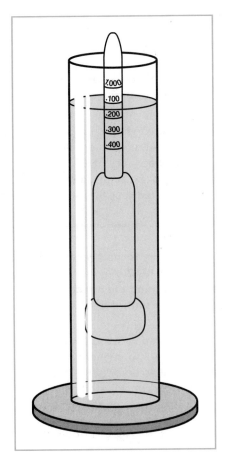

FIGURE 10-2 Urinometer. (From Doucette, L. J. [1997]. *Mathematics for the Clinical Laboratory* [p. 188]. Philadelphia: W.B. Saunders.)

float has an etched scale that ranges from 0.000 to 0.030. As the float is placed in the urine, it rises to the top of the urine specimen. The specific gravity reading is determined by the intersection of the scale with the bottom of the meniscus of the urine. When the urinometer is placed in deionized water, the measurement should be 1.000. As part of the laboratory's quality assurance plan, the urinometer is checked with deionized water before use with patient specimens to ensure that it is properly calibrated. If the urinometer does not read 1.000 with deionized water, all patient specimens must be adjusted correspondingly to ensure accurate results.

The refractometer, or total solids (TS) meter (see Figure 10-3), measures specific gravity indirectly by the refractive index of the urine. The refractive index is a ratio of the velocity of light in air to the velocity of light in solution. The angle at which the light passes through the solution is converted mathematically into units of specific gravity. Only one drop of urine is required with a refractometer. The refractometer can be calibrated with deionized water to read 1.000.

PROBLEMS

A urinometer used in a physician's office laboratory is checked with deionized water to determine if it is calibrated. The reading is 1.003. A quality control specimen with a specific gravity of 1.022 also is measured using the urinometer. What adjustments or corrections must be made to the quality control result and all other control or patient results?

The specific gravity of deionized water, as measured with a urinometer, should be 1.000. In this problem the measurement is 1.003. All subsequent results (for quality controls and patients) must be adjusted for the inaccuracy of +0.003 in the reading. The quality control specimen's specific gravity must be adjusted by subtracting 0.003 from the measured reading. Therefore, the corrected specific gravity for the quality control specimen is 1.019.

A urinometer used in a physician's office laboratory is checked with deionized water to determine if it is calibrated. The reading is 1.002. A quality control specimen with a specific gravity of 1.026 also is measured using the urinometer. What adjustments or corrections must be made to the quality control result and all other control or patient results?

The specific gravity of deionized water, as measured with a urinometer, should be 1.000. In this problem the measurement is 1.002. All subsequent results (for quality controls and patients) must be adjusted for the inaccuracy of +0.002 in the reading. The quality control specimen's specific gravity must be adjusted by subtracting 0.002 point from the measured reading. Therefore, the corrected specific gravity for the quality control specimen is 1.024.

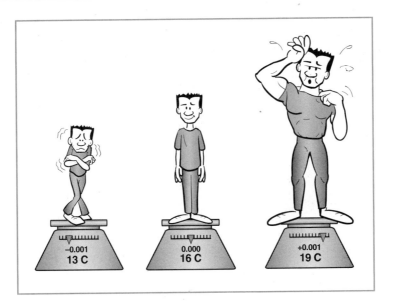

Correction for Temperature

A consideration when using a urinometer, but not a refractometer, is that temperature will influence specific gravity measurements. A urinometer is calibrated by the manufacturer to read 0.000 with deionized water at a temperature of 16°C (about 60°F). For every 3 degrees higher than the calibration temperature, 0.001 must be added to the specific gravity reading. For every 3 degrees lower, 0.001 must be subtracted from the reading. The calibrated temperature is the temperature of urine at room temperature. Urine specimens taken directly from a refrigerator or freshly voided have very different temperatures. The temperatures of these specimens should be established and the specific gravity measurements adjusted if a urinometer is used.

PROBLEMS

As part of a physical examination at a doctor's office, a freshly voided urine specimen obtained from a patient was given to the medical assistant for urinalysis. The medical assistant immediately performed a specific gravity test using a urinometer and obtained a measurement of 1.018. The assistant noted that the urine was quite warm and determined that its temperature was 36.5°C. What is the correct specific gravity reading?

Since specific gravity is affected by temperature, the specific gravity measurement of the urine must be corrected to reflect the higher temperature of the urine. Freshly voided urine will have a temperature much higher than urine at room temperature. Add 0.001 for every 3 degrees higher than the calibration temperature.

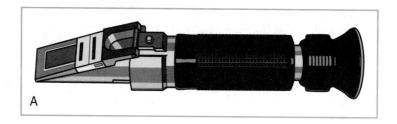

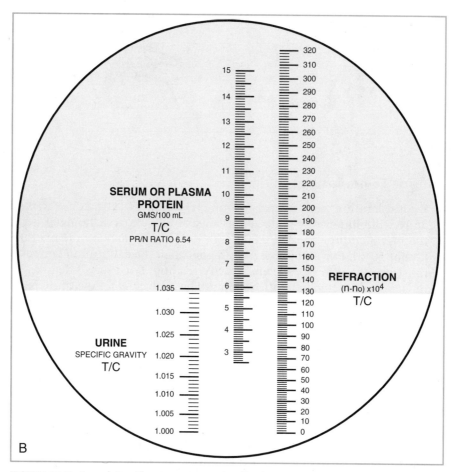

FIGURE 10-3 *A* and *B*, refractometer scale. (From *Instructions for Use and Care of the Leica TS Meter*. Leica Optical Products Division, Buffalo, NY, with permission. Courtesy of Leica, Inc.)

Calibration temperature = 16°C
Urine temperature = 36.5°C

Then 36.5 − 16 = 20.5°C (the difference between the calibrated temperature and the specimen's temperature).

Divide the temperature difference by 3 (because of the factor of 3 degrees)

$$\frac{20.5}{3} = 6.8$$

Multiply the result by 0.001 to obtain the "correction factor":

6.8 × 0.001 = 0.007

To correct for the warmer temperature, add 0.007 to 1.018:

1.018 + 0.007 = 1.025

The corrected specific gravity for this specimen is 1.025.

In a small, short-staffed health clinic, the morning urine specimens were placed in a refrigerator until the medical assistant began to analyze them 45 minutes later. When the medical assistant removed the specimens from the refrigerator and began to analyze them, she found that the first specimen had a specific gravity by urinometer of 1.015. She noted that the urine was pale yellow. Its temperature was 7.2°C. What is the true specific gravity of this specimen?

Because the urine was refrigerated, its temperature was below the standard temperature of 16°C. The urinometer measurement must be corrected by subtracting 0.001 for every 3 degrees below this standard temperature.

$$16°C − 7.2°C = 8.8°C$$
$$\frac{8.8}{3} = 3$$
$$3 × 0.001 = 0.003$$
$$1.015 − 0.003 = 1.012$$

The corrected specific gravity for this specimen is 1.012.

Early one morning, a renal patient arrived at the doctor's office to drop off a 24 hour urine specimen that was to be analyzed in a reference laboratory. The laboratory required at least 30 mL of the specimen to be shipped frozen on dry ice. While the medical assistant was processing the specimen, the doctor examined the patient. Thirty minutes after the medical assistant had placed a 50 mL aliquot of the urine in the laboratory freezer, the doctor asked if a urinalysis could be performed before the aliquot was shipped to the reference laboratory. The medical assistant immediately removed the aliquot from the freezer and began to perform the urinalysis. The aliquot was cold but not yet frozen. A specific gravity of 1.010 was measured by the urinometer, and the urine was straw-colored and clear. The doctor questioned the specific gravity value because it did not match the light appearance of the urine. The medical assistant realized that the sample was still quite cold and determined its temperature to be 2°C. What is the patient's correct urine specific gravity?

Since the standard temperature is 16°C, subtract the measured temperature from this standard:

16 − 2 = 14°C

Next, divide 14 by the factor of 3:

$$\frac{14}{3} = 4.6$$

Next, multiply 5 by 0.001:

5 × 0.001 = 1.005

Finally, subtract 0.005 from the specific gravity reading of 1.010 to obtain the correct specific gravity reading:

1.010 − 0.005 = 1.005

The patient's urine specific gravity is really 1.005, not 1.010, which fits its straw-colored appearance.

Correction for Protein

Both the urinometer and the refractometer must be corrected if large quantities of protein (1 g/dL or more) are present in the urine. Protein is a very high molecular weight compound that will increase the density of the urine by 0.003 for every 1 g/dL of protein. Protein is not normally found in the urine because it cannot pass through the glomerular membrane. When the integrity of the glomerulus is compromised due to injury or disease, protein molecules can pass through the glomerulus and appear in the urine. The purpose of measuring the specific gravity of the urine is to determine the concentrating ability of the kidneys, which depends primarily on the renal tubules. The presence of large amounts of protein (1 g/dL or more) in the urine will falsely increase the specific gravity and result in erroneous assessment of the kidneys.

PROBLEMS

A urinalysis was performed on a urine specimen that contained 2.5 g/dL of protein. The specific gravity by refractometer was 1.026. What is the corrected specific gravity for this sample?

Each 1 g/dL of protein falsely elevates the specific gravity by 0.003. Since the urine contains 3 g/dL of protein, the amount to be subtracted is 2.5 × 0.003 = 0.008.

Corrected specific gravity = 1.026 − 0.008 = 1.016

Therefore, the specific gravity of the sample that reflects the concentrating ability of the kidneys is 1.016.

A urinalysis was performed on a urine specimen that contained 1.2 g/dL of protein. The specific gravity by refractometer was 1.015. What is the corrected specific gravity for this sample?

Each 1 g/dL of protein falsely elevates the specific gravity by 0.003. Since the urine contains 1.2 g/dL of protein, the amount to be subtracted is 1.2 × 0.003 = 0.004. Therefore, 0.004 is subtracted from 1.015 to obtain the corrected specific gravity:

$$1.015 - 0.004 = 1.011$$

The true specific gravity of this urine is 1.011.

Correction for Glucose

Glucose, like protein, is a high molecular weight compound. When it is present in large quantities (1 g/dL or more), the specific gravity of the urine will be increased by 0.004 for every 1 g/dL of glucose. As with protein, increased glucose levels do not reflect the concentrating ability of the renal tubules. The effect of 1 g/dL or more of glucose must be subtracted from the specific gravity to obtain an accurate measurement.

PROBLEMS

A urine specimen has a glucose concentration of 1 g/dL and a specific gravity of 1.018. What is the corrected specific gravity?

For each 1 g/dL of glucose, the specific gravity is elevated by 0.004. The corrected specific gravity is:

$$\text{Corrected specific gravity} = 1.018 - (0.004)(1)$$
$$= 1.018 - 0.004$$
$$= 1.014$$

Therefore, the corrected specific gravity is 1.014.

A urine specimen had a glucose concentration of 2.5 g/dL and a measured specific gravity of 1.032. What is its corrected specific gravity?

For every 1 g/dL of glucose in a urine specimen, 0.004 must be subtracted from its measured specific gravity. Therefore:

$$1.032 - (0.004)(2.5) = X$$
$$1.032 - 0.010 = X$$
$$X = 1.022$$

Thus, the corrected specific gravity is 1.022.

EXAMPLE PROBLEMS

This section is designed to be useful to both the student and the health care practitioner. Students can use the example problems in order to master the material. The health care practitioner can use these problems as templates for performing laboratory calculations. Find an example problem similar to the problem that you need to solve and substitute into the equation the numbers appropriate to your calculation.

1. **Q** **A urine specimen collected over 6 hours has a volume of 575 mL and a potassium value of 35 mEq/L. What is the potassium concentration in this specimen?**

   A This problem is solved using ratio and proportion. *Note:* the collection volume in milliliters must be expressed in liters to keep the units comparable.

   $$\frac{35 \text{ mEq}}{1 \text{ L}} = \frac{X \text{ mEq}}{0.575 \text{ L}}$$

   Cross-multiplying the equation yields:
   $$(35)(0.575) = (1)(X)$$
   $$20.1 = X.$$

   Therefore, this 575 mL of urine contains 20 mEq of potassium.

2. **Q** **For the patient in example problem 1, what is the urine potassium concentration in mEq/6 hr?**

   A Whenever a urine specimen is collected in less than 24 hours, the results can be recorded as concentration per volume collected, concentration per time collected, or concentration extrapolated to a 24 hour collection period. The results for concentration per volume collected and concentration per time collected are similar; only the units are different. In this problem, 20 mEq of potassium in 575 mL of urine was collected in 6 hours. The result can be recorded as 17 mEq/575 mL or as 17 mEq/6 hr. Both results are equivalent.

3. **Q** **A 12 hour urine specimen with a volume of 750 mL was collected for sodium analysis. The result is 95 mEq/L. What is the result in terms of quantity per total volume?**

   A The patient's urine volume is 750 mL and the quantity of sodium is 95 mEq/L. Using ratio and proportion, the amount of sodium found in the 750 mL of specimen can be calculated:

$$\frac{95 \text{ mEq}}{1000 \text{ mL}} = \frac{X \text{ mEq}}{750 \text{ mL}}$$

Cross-multiplying the equation yields:

(X)(1000) = (95)(750)

(X)(1000) = 71,250

X = 71 mEq/750 mL.

4. Q **What is the patient's sodium value in terms of mEq/12 hr?**

A Since the urine was collected over 12 hours and the volume collected within that time period is 750 mL, the results of 71 mEq/750 mL and 71 mEq/12 hr are equivalent. Therefore, the sodium value in terms of mEq/12 hr is 71 mEq/12 hr.

5. Q **A 24 hour urine specimen was collected for a creatinine clearance test. The urine volume is 1800 mL, the plasma creatinine value is 2.4 mg/dL, and the creatinine clearance test result is 167 mg/dL. What is the patient's uncorrected creatinine clearance value?**

A The formula for determining clearance is:

$$\frac{UV}{P}$$

Where:

U = urine concentration in mg/dL of the analyte cleared

V = volume of urine in mL/min

P = plasma concentration of analyte in mg/dL

To determine the volume of urine in mL/min, multiply the number of hours of collection by 60 to determine the length of time in minutes:

24 × 60 = 1440 minutes.

Next, divide the quantity of urine collected by the number of minutes to obtain the quantity in mL/min:

$$\frac{1800 \text{ mL}}{2400 \text{ min}} = 1.25 \text{ mL/min}.$$

Next, substitute into the clearance equation the data that are known:

$$\text{Clearance (mL/min)} = \frac{(167 \text{ mg/dL})(1.25 \text{ mL/min})}{2.4 \text{ mg/dL}}$$

$$= 87 \text{ mL/min}.$$

6. Q **A 6 hour creatinine clearance test was performed on a urine specimen with a volume of 415 mL. The urine creatinine and plasma creatinine concentrations are 50 mg/dL and 2.5 mg/dL, respectively. What is the patient's creatinine clearance?**

A To answer this question, first convert the amount of urine excreted in 6 hours to mL/min excreted. In 6 hours there are 360 minutes. By dividing the volume of urine excreted, 415 mL, by 360, the amount of urine volume per mL/min can be calculated. The result is 1.25 mL/min. Using the clearance formula, the creatinine clearance can be calculated:

$$\text{Clearance (mL/min)} = \frac{(50 \text{ mg/dL})(1.25 \text{ mL/min})}{2.5 \text{ mg/dL}}$$

$$= 25.$$

Therefore, the creatinine clearance is 25 mL/min.

7. **Q** **A creatinine clearance test was performed on a 95-year-old woman who was 4 feet 11 inches tall and weighed 105 pounds. The 24 hour urine specimen has a volume of 1050 mL and a creatinine concentration of 125 mg/dL. The plasma creatinine concentration is 1.8 mg/dL. What is the patient's corrected creatinine clearance?**

A The clearance formula is based on the average height and weight of men. For any person with a body size that is significantly smaller or larger, the clearance formula should be adjusted accordingly. The nomogram can be used to adjust the clearance formula. Based on average male height and weight, the body surface area of the average male is 1.73 m². The clearance formula is slightly modified to correct for size differences. The corrected clearance formula is:

$$\frac{UV}{P} \times \frac{1.73 \text{ m}^2}{\text{body surface area of patient from nomogram}}$$

Using the nomogram in Figure 10-1, determine the patient's body surface area by drawing a line from the point indicating 4 feet 11 inches on the height scale to 105 pounds on the weight scale. The point of intersection on the body surface area scale is 1.29 m². Next, determine the patient's rate of urine flow in mL/min by dividing 1050 mL by the number of minutes in 24 hours, or 1440 minutes. Next, use the clearance formula to determine the patient's clearance:

$$\text{Clearance} = \frac{(125 \text{ mg/dL}) (0.73 \text{ mL/min})}{1.8 \text{ mg/dL}} \times \frac{1.73 \text{ m}^2}{1.29 \text{ m}^2}$$

$$= 50.7 \times 1.34$$

$$= 68 \text{ mL/min}.$$

8. **Q** **A creatinine clearance test is performed on a professional football player. The patient is 6 feet 6 inches tall and weighs 345 pounds. A 24 hour urine sample with a volume of 2500 mL was**

obtained. The urine creatinine concentration is 175 mg/dL, and the serum creatinine concentration is 3.5 mg/dL. What is the patient's corrected creatinine clearance?

A To solve this problem, first convert the total volume of urine collected into the amount collected in mL/min. This is accomplished by dividing 2500 mL (the amount collected) by 1440 (the number of minutes in 24 hours), yielding a result of 1.74 mL/min. Next, using the nomogram in Figure 10-1, determine the patient's body surface area. Draw a line between the patient's height (6 feet 6 inches) and the patient's weight (345 pounds). The line intersects the surface area scale at 2.64 m². Finally, substitute all data into the corrected clearance formula:

$$\text{Corrected clearance} = \frac{(175\ \text{mg/dL})(1.74\ \text{mL/min})}{3.5\ \text{mg/dL}} \times \frac{1.73\ \text{m}^2}{2.64\ \text{m}^2}$$
$$= (87\ \text{mL/min})(0.655)$$
$$= 57.0\ \text{mL/min.}$$

9. **Q** **A freshly voided urine specimen is immediately brought to the laboratory for a urinalysis. The specific gravity by urinometer is 1.008. The medical assistant notices that the urine is warm and determines its temperature to be 27°C. What is the corrected specific gravity reading?**

A The density or specific gravity measured by urinometer is temperature dependent. The colder a liquid, the higher its density. This is demonstrated by the fact that ice is denser than water. If urine is warmer or colder than the calibrated temperature of 16°C, then the specific gravity must be adjusted for the temperature difference by subtracting 0.001 from the reading for every 3°C below 16°C and adding 0.001 for every 3°C above 16°C. To determine the amount that must be adjusted, first subtract the urine temperature from the calibration temperature of 16°C, ignoring any negative signs:

   16°C − 27°C = 11°C.

Next, divide 11°C by the factor 3:

   11 ÷ 3 = 3.6.

The result, 3.6, is rounded to 4.

Next, multiply 0.001 by 4:

   0.001 × 4 = 0.004.

Add 0.004 to the specific gravity reading obtained:

   1.008 + 0.004 = 1.012.

Therefore, the corrected specific gravity is 1.012.

10. **Q** A patient submits a urine specimen to the doctor's office laboratory for analysis. The specific gravity is measured using a refractometer, and a result of 1.020 is obtained. Since the urine is
warm (32°C), what is the patient's correct specific gravity?

   A The patient's specific gravity reading is not changed because the test
is performed using a refractometer. Urinometers are temperature sensitive, and readings above or below the calibrated temperature of
16°C must be adjusted. No adjustment is necessary with a refractometer because it is not temperature sensitive. Therefore, the patient's
urine specific gravity remains at 1.020.

11. **Q** A nurse removes a urine specimen from the refrigerator and performs a urinalysis. The specific gravity, determined by urinometer, is 1.010. The nurse notices that the urine is straw-colored
and decides that its appearance does not match its specific gravity. The temperature of the urine is 5.0°C. What is its correct specific gravity?

   A The specific gravity, or density, of urine increases with cold. Urinometers are calibrated to be used at approximately 16°C. For every 3°C
less, 0.001 must be subtracted from the specific gravity reading. To determine the amount that should be subtracted, first subtract the urine
temperature from the calibrated temperature:
   16.0°C − 5.0°C = 11°C difference.
   Next, divide the difference, 11, by the factor of 3:
   11 ÷ 3 = 3.6 or 4.
   Next, multiply the factor, 4, by 0.001:
   4 × 0.001 = 0.004.
   Finally, subtract 0.004 from 1.010:
   1.010 − 0.004 = 1.006.
   The correct specific gravity is 1.006.

12. **Q** A urinalysis is performed on a urine specimen that contains
3 g/dL of protein. The specific gravity, measured by a refractometer, is 1.025. What is the correct specific gravity for this urine?

   A Protein levels of 1 g/dL or more will falsely elevate the specific gravity
reading by refractometer or urinometer. For every gram of protein,
the specific gravity will be elevated by 0.001. Since the urine contains
a protein concentration of 3 g/dL, the specific gravity is falsely elevated by 0.003. Subtracting 0.003 from the obtained specific gravity of
1.025 results in the correct specific gravity of 1.022.

13. **Q** **A urine specimen from a diabetic patient has a glucose level of 3.0 g/dL. The specific gravity of the patient's urine by urinometer is 1.030. What is the patient's correct specific gravity?**

   A For each 1 g/dL of glucose present in a urine specimen, the specific gravity is falsely elevated by 0.004. Since the urine contains a glucose concentration of 3 g/dL, the effect is a false increase in specific gravity of 0.012. When 0.012 is subtracted from the specific gravity of 1.030, the result, 1.018, is the correct specific gravity.

PRACTICE PROBLEMS

Solve the following problems to further master the material. Answers and explanations to some problems can be found in a separate section at the back of the book.

Given the following analyte concentrations, urine collection times, and volumes, express them in terms of concentration per volume of collection.

1. Sodium concentration of 25 mEq/L, collected over 12 hours, 950 mL volume.
2. Glucose concentration of 65 mg/dL, collected over 24 hours, 1350 mL volume.
3. Creatinine concentration of 525 mg/dL, collected over 24 hours, 1345 mL volume.

Express the following in terms of concentration per time.

4. Creatinine value of 1000 mg/2240 mL collected over 24 hours.
5. Potassium result of 40 mEq/734 mL collected over 12 hours.

Calculate both the uncorrected and corrected creatinine clearance values for the following problems.

Female patient: height 5 feet 6 inches, weight 140 pounds, urine creatinine 188 mg/dL, collection time 24 hours, plasma creatinine 1.8 mg/dL, urine volume 2432 mL.

6. Uncorrected creatinine clearance.
7. Corrected creatinine clearance.

Male patient: height 5 feet 11 inches, weight 165 pounds, urine creatinine 117 mg/dL, collection time 24 hours, plasma creatinine 2.3 mg/dL, urine volume 1690 mL.

8. Uncorrected creatinine clearance.
9. Corrected creatinine clearance.

Correct the following specific gravity results obtained with a urinometer.

10. Specific gravity 1.027, urine temperature 4°C.
11. Specific gravity 1.025, urine temperature 10°C.
12. Specific gravity 1.013, urine temperature 32°C.
13. Specific gravity 1.004, urine temperature 25°C.
14. Specific gravity 1.025, urine protein concentration of 2.0 g/dL.
15. Specific gravity 1.032, urine protein concentration of 4.0 g/dL.
16. Specific gravity 1.038, urine glucose concentration of 3.0 g/dL.
17. Specific gravity 1.029, urine glucose concentration of 2.0 g/dL.

BIBLIOGRAPHY

Anderson, S., and Cockayne, S. *Clinical Chemistry: Concepts and Applications*. W.B. Saunders Company, Philadelphia, 1993.

Burtis, C. A., and Ashwood, E. R. *Tietz Textbook of Clinical Chemistry*, 3rd ed. W.B. Saunders Company, Philadelphia, 1999.

Strasinger, S. *Urinalysis and Body Fluids*, 3rd ed. F.A. Davis Company, Philadelphia, 1994.

CHAPTER 11

Hematology and Immunohematology Laboratories

INTRODUCTION

Red Blood Cell Indices

Hematology is the study of the cells within the blood. These include the white blood cells (WBCs), platelets, and the cells occurring in the largest quantity, the red blood cells (RBCs). The RBCs carry oxygen from the lungs to the tissues and carbon dioxide from the tissues back to the lungs, where it is exhaled. The oxygen is carried by a hemoglobin molecule. The quantity of hemoglobin can be determined by hematology instruments. Some instruments are simple and measure only hemoglobin, while other instruments are complex and measure other hematology parameters as well, such as the WBC count, the RBC count, and the hemoglobin concentration of a sample. If the hemoglobin concentration is low, the oxygen-carrying capacity of the RBC is decreased as well. This leads to the condition called *anemia*. The most common cause of anemia is iron deficiency. Iron is vital to the structure of the hemoglobin molecule, and if the iron concentration is low, the hemoglobin concentration will be reduced.

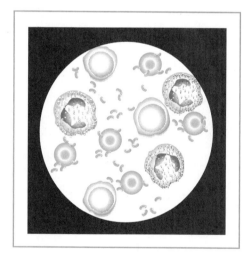
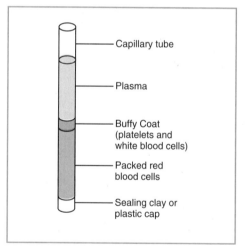

Another common hematology test is the hematocrit. This is the ratio of the blood cells to plasma expressed as a percentage. Normally, in healthy individuals, the hematocrit has a value of 37–52%, meaning that approximately half of the whole blood in the body is made up of cellular components, while the remainder consists of liquid plasma. If the RBC concentration is decreased, the hematocrit will be decreased. If a person is anemic, the hemoglobin and hematocrit will both be decreased.

The size of the RBC is important in the treatment of anemia. Some forms of anemia cause the RBC to be smaller than normal; others cause it to be larger. The relationship between size, hemoglobin, and hematocrit was determined mathematically by Maxwell M. Wintrobe in the 1920s. Three formulas were developed to describe RBC morphology and to aid in the classification of anemia. The first is the *mean corpuscular volume (MCV)*. The MCV describes the average volume or size of the RBC in femtoliters (fL) or its equivalent, cubic microns (μ^3), and is calculated by the following formula:

$$\frac{MCV}{(fL \text{ or } \mu^3)} = \frac{\text{Hematocrit (\%)} \times 10}{\text{RBC count (millions per } \mu L)}$$

The normal range for MCV is 80–96 fL. MCV values below 80 fL suggest that RBCs are smaller than normal, while MCV values above 96 fL suggest that RBCs are larger than normal.

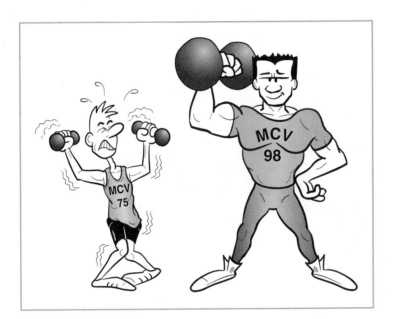

PROBLEMS

Calculate the MCV of a sample if the hematocrit is 42% and the RBC count is 5 (millions per µL).

Use the formula to calculate MCV:

$$MCV = \frac{HCT \times 10}{RBC \text{ count}} = \frac{42 \times 10}{5} = 84 \text{ fL}$$

The MCV of this sample is 84 fL.

Calculate the MCV of a sample if the hematocrit is 30% and the RBC count is 4.5 (millions per µL).

Use the formula to calculate MCV:

$$\text{MCV} = \frac{\text{HCT} \times 10}{\text{RBC count}} = \frac{30 \times 10}{4.5} = 67 \text{ fL}$$

The MCV of this sample is 67 fL.

The second formula is the *mean corpuscular hemoglobin (MCH)*. As its name implies it represents the average amount of hemoglobin present in the individual RBC in micromicrograms (µµg) or their equivalent, picograms (pg), significant to the nearest tenth. It is calculated by the following formula:

$$\text{MCH (µµg or pg)} = \frac{\text{Hemoglobin (g/dL)} \times 10}{\text{RBC count (millions per µL)}}$$

The normal range for MCH is 27–31 pg.

PROBLEMS

Calculate the MCH of a patient with a hemoglobin concentration of 17 g/dL and a RBC count of 6.5 million/µL.

Use the formula to calculate MCH:

$$\frac{\text{Hb} \times 10}{\text{RBC count}} = \frac{17 \times 10}{6.5} = \frac{170}{6.5} = 26 \text{ pg}$$

Therefore, the MCH for this patient is 26 pg.

Calculate the MCH of a patient with a hemoglobin concentration of 14 g/dL and a RBC count of 4.3 million/µL.

Use the formula to calculate MCH:

$$\frac{\text{Hb} \times 10}{\text{RBC count}} = \frac{14 \times 10}{4.3} = \frac{140}{4.3} = 33 \text{ pg}$$

The third formula is the mean corpuscular hemoglobin concentration (MCMC). It expresses the ratio of the hemoglobin to the hematocrit in percentage terms significant to the nearest tenth. The MCHC represents the average hemoglobin content in the patient's RBC population.

$$\text{MCHC} = \frac{\text{Hemoglobin (g/dL)} \times 100}{\text{Hematocrit (\%)}}$$

The normal range for MCHC is 32–36%.

PROBLEMS

Calculate the MCHC of a patient with a hemoglobin concentration of 10 g/dL and a hematocrit of 32%.

Use the formula to calculate MCHC:

$$\frac{\text{Hb g/dL} \times 100}{32\%} = \frac{10 \times 100}{32} = \frac{1000}{32} = 31\%$$

Calculate the MCHC of a patient with a hemoglobin concentration of 15 g/dL and a hematocrit of 45%.

Use the formula to calculate MCHC:

$$\frac{\text{Hb g/dL} \times 100}{45\%} = \frac{15 \times 100}{45} = \frac{1500}{45} = 33\%$$

Cell Counting by the Hemacytometer Method

The majority of RBC, WBC, and platelet counts are performed by automated hematology analyzers. Occasionally, the count may be too low for the instrument to count the cells accurately. In these instances, cells must be counted with the aid of a microscope using a counting chamber called a *hemacytometer* (Figure 11-1). The most common hemacytometer used in clinical hematology is the Neubauer hemocytometer. It consists of two identical counting chambers. Each chamber contains an etched grid with a total surface area of 9 mm². The chambers are identical so that a sample can be counted in duplicate using the same hemocytometer. The counts from both chambers should be within 10% of each other to ensure accuracy. Whole blood is most commonly diluted using the Unopette system, which consists of a collection pipette and a reservoir filled with diluent. The types of diluent and the dilution performed vary with the type of cell counted. A small amount of sample is allowed to flow between the coverslip and the hemacytometer chamber. The distance between the coverslip and the surface of the hemacytometer is 0.1 mm.

An older method still in use for fluid cell counts is the manual dilution technique using Thoma pipettes. Using a pipetter device, blood is aspirated to the calibrated mark followed by stain until the Thoma pipette is filled. The dilutions obtained with the Unopette and Thoma pipette are the same for all cell types.

Figure 11-1 is a schematic of a Neubauer hemacytometer grid, with each square numbered 1–9. The hemacytometer is divided into nine large squares. WBCs are counted in the four corner squares (squares 1, 3, 7, and 9) while platelets and RBCs are counted in the central square (square 5). The large squares are further divided into 16 smaller squares to facilitate ease of counting the WBCs. The center square is divided into 25 small squares. Each of the 25 small squares is further divided into 16 smaller squares for RBC and platelet counting.

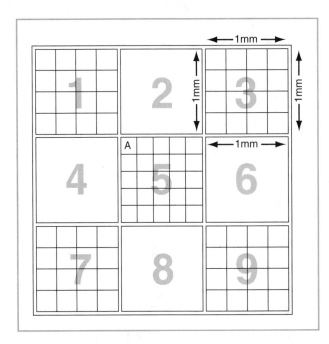

FIGURE 11-1 Neubauer hemo-cytometer. (From Doucette, L. J. [1997]. *Mathematics for the Clinical Laboratory* [p. 205]. Philadelphia: W.B. Saunders Company.)

WBC Count

When the WBC count is abnormally elevated or decreased, or when the quantity of WBCs in fluid such as cerebrospinal fluid or joint fluid must be determined, the hemacytometer method is used to perform the total WBC count. Using either the Thoma pipette or the Unopette system for WBCs, a $1/20$ dilution is usually used for the total WBC count. The Unopette system designed for both platelets and WBCs yields a $1/100$ dilution. Occasionally, a $1/10$ dilution is performed if the WBC count is abnormally decreased. WBCs are counted using high power or 400× magnification in each of the 16 smaller squares contained in each of the 4 corner squares. The area of each large square is 1 mm², and the depth is 0.1 mm. Therefore, the volume of each large square is 0.1 mm³ (volume = area × depth).

The formula used to calculate the number of cells per cubic millimeter is:

$$\text{Cells/mm}^3 = \frac{\text{Cells counted} \times \text{depth factor} \times \text{dilution factor}}{\text{total area counted}}$$

where:

    area counted = number of large squares counted
    depth factor = reciprocal of depth $[1/(1/10)] = 10$
 dilution factor = reciprocal of dilution

PROBLEM

A WBC count was performed on a sample that was abnormally decreased below the linearity of the automated cell counter. A ¹/₁₀ dilution was performed, and all WBCs in each of the four corner squares of both grids of the hemacytometer were counted. A total of 120 WBCs were counted. What is the total WBC count?

In this problem, all eight squares were counted; therefore, the area counted is 8. The dilution factor is 10 since a ¹/₁₀ dilution was performed. Substituting into the formula for cell counting, the following equation is derived:

$$\text{WBCs/mm}^3 = \frac{120 \text{ WBCs counted} \times 10 \text{ (depth factor)} \times 10 \text{ (dilution factor)}}{8 \text{ (total area counted)}}$$

$$= 1500$$

For many WBC counts, the dilution performed is ¹/₂₀ and all WBCs within the four corner squares are counted. Therefore, within the volume in one large square is the number of WBCs per ¹/₂₀₀ mm³ of blood (0.1 mm³ × ¹/₂₀). This amount is multiplied by the number of squares counted (four). Thus, the typical WBC count quantifies the number of WBCs per 50 mm³ (¹/₂₀₀ × 4) of blood.

The factor of 50 can be used to quickly calculate the WBC count using a hemacytometer. Simply multiply the total number of cells counted by 50 to yield the total WBC count/mm³.

> **Note** This factor of 50 can be used *only* if the dilution performed is ¹/₂₀ and all WBCs in the four large corner squares are counted.

In the formula used to calculate the factor:

Factor = 1/area × depth factor × dilution factor
Area counted = number of large squares counted
Depth factor = reciprocal of depth [1/(¹/₁₀)] = 10
Dilution factor = reciprocal of dilution = [1/(¹/₂₀)] = 20

Therefore, the factor is:

$$\frac{1}{4} \times 10 \times 20 = 50$$

PROBLEMS

A WBC count was performed using a hemacytometer and a ¹/₂₀ dilution. A total of 230 WBCs were counted in the four large squares. Using the factor method, what is the total WBC count?

The factor $= \frac{1}{4} \times 10 \times 20 = 50$

Multiply the number of cells counted by the factor of 50:

50 × 230 = 11,500

Therefore, the WBC count is 11,500/mm³. WBC counts may be reported in one of three ways. Since 1 mm³ is equal to 1 µL, the count may be reported as 11,500/µL. In addition, 1 fL is equal to 1000 µL, so many laboratories may report the count as 11.5 × 10⁹/L.

A WBC count was performed using a hemacytometer and a ¹/₂₀ dilution. A total of 185 WBCs were counted in the four large squares. Using the factor method, what is the total WBC count?

Multiply the number of cells counted by the factor of 50:

50 × 185 = 9250

Therefore, the white blood cell count is 9250/mm³.

RBC Count

Since there are so many more RBCs than WBCs, the cells are diluted ¹/₂₀₀. The RBCs are counted in the four corner squares and the center square within the large central square. Each of these small squares is subdivided into 16 smaller squares to make counting easier. Figure 11-2 is an enlargement of one of the center squares to aid in visualization of the 16 small squares. Therefore, there is a total of 80 squares in which the RBCs are counted. Each of the 25 small squares within the large central square is 0.04 mm² (0.2 mm × 0.2 mm). Because five of these squares are counted, the total area counted is 0.04 × 5 or 0.2 mm². As in WBC counting, a factor can be calculated and used to quantify RBCs easily.

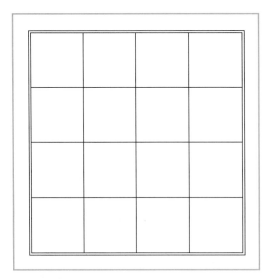

FIGURE 11-2 Enlargement of square A in the Neubauer hemocytometer. (From Doucette, L. J. [1997]. *Mathematics for the Clinical Laboratory* [p. 206]. Philadelphia: W.B. Saunders Company.)

In the formula to calculate the factor for RBC counts:

Factor = 1/area × depth factor × dilution factor
Area counted = area of small squares counted = 0.2 mm²
Depth factor = reciprocal of depth [1/($\frac{1}{10}$)] = 10
Dilution factor = reciprocal of dilution = [1/($\frac{1}{200}$)] = 200

Therefore, the factor is:

$$\frac{1}{0.2} \times 10 \times 200 = 10,000$$

PROBLEMS

An RBC count was performed on a sample that was diluted $\frac{1}{200}$. A total of 552 RBCs were counted in the 80 small squares used for RBC counts. What is the total RBC count in terms of 10^6/mm³?

Use the factor method to solve this problem; the factor is 10,000. Since 552 cells were counted, the RBC count is:

10,000 × 552 = 5,520,000 or 5.52 × 10^6/mm³

An RBC count was performed on a sample that was diluted $\frac{1}{200}$. A total of 381 RBCs were counted in the 80 small squares used for RBC counts. What is the total RBC count in terms of 10^6/mm³?

Use the factor method to solve this problem; the factor is equal to 10,000. Since 381 cells were counted, the RBC count is:

10,000 × 381 = 3,810,000 or 3.81 × 10^6/mm³

Platelet Count

Platelets are small fragments of cells found in the bone marrow called *megakaryocytes*. Platelets function in the initial phase of the coagulation process. All 25 squares in the central square of the hemacytometer are used to count platelets. Remember that within each of the 25 squares are 16 smaller squares, so the total number of squares counted for platelets is 400. Since each of the 25 squares has an area of 0.04 mm² and all 25 squares are counted, the total area counted is 1 mm² (0.04 × 25). A $\frac{1}{100}$ dilution is performed on the whole blood for platelet counting. Like WBC and RBC counts, platelet counts can have a calculated factor.
    In the formula for the factor for platelets:

Factor = 1/area × depth factor × dilution factor
Area counted = area of small squares counted
Depth factor = reciprocal of depth [1/($\frac{1}{10}$)] = 10
Dilution factor = reciprocal of dilution = [1/($\frac{1}{100}$)] = 100

Therefore, the factor is:

$$\frac{1}{1.0} \times 10 \times 100 = 1000$$

PROBLEMS

A platelet count was performed using a ¹⁄₁₀₀ dilution and counting all platelets found in the 400 small squares of the central square in the hemacytometer. A total of 350 platelets were counted. Using the factor method, what is the platelet count?

The factor for platelets is 1000. Since 350 platelets were counted, then the total platelet count is:

350 × **1000** = 350,000/mm³

A platelet count was performed using a ¹⁄₁₀₀ dilution and counting all platelets found in the 400 small squares of the central square in the hemacytometer. A total of 74 platelets were counted. Using the factor method, what is the platelet count?

The factor for platelets is 1000. Since 74 platelets were counted, the total platelet count is:

74 × **1000** = 74,000/mm³

Reticulocyte Count

Slide Method

Reticulocytes are slightly immature RBCs that usually cannot be distinguished from mature RBCs (erythrocytes) on a Wright-stained smear. Unlike mature RBCs, reticulocytes contain small clumps of ribosomal RNA. This ribosomal RNA can be stained with a supravital stain such as brilliant cresyl blue or new methylene blue so that the reticulocytes can be distinguished from mature RBCs. When stained with supravital stains, ribosomal RNA looks like blue strands or granules in the RBC. To perform a reticulocyte count, equal amounts of blood and stain are mixed and incubated at room temperature for 10 minutes. A smear is made of the mixture and allowed to air dry. Using the oil immersion lens, 1000 mature RBCs are counted consecutively, and the number of reticulocytes found among the 1000 mature cells is noted. A reticulocyte count is a percentage count of the number of reticulocytes per 1000 mature RBCs. It is calculated using the following formula:

$$\% \text{ Reticulocytes} = \frac{\text{\# Reticulocytes counted per 1000 erythrocytes}}{1000} \times 100$$

PROBLEMS

A reticulocyte count was performed, and 24 reticulocytes were counted per 1000 erythrocytes. What is the reticulocyte percentage?

$$\% \text{ Reticulocytes} = \frac{\text{\# Reticulocytes counted per 1000 erythrocytes}}{1000} \times 100$$

$$= \frac{24}{1000} \times 100 = 2.4\%$$

A reticulocyte count was performed, and 15 reticulocytes were counted per 1000 erythrocytes. What is the reticulocyte percentage?

$$\% \text{ Reticulocytes} = \frac{\text{\# Reticulocytes counted per 1000 erythrocytes}}{1000} \times 100$$

$$= \frac{15}{1000} \times 100 = 1.5\%$$

Miller Disc Method

Another method of counting reticulocytes involves the use of a special glass insert for the eyepiece lens of a microscope. The glass insert fits into one of the eyepiece lenses and has a central large square (1) within which is a smaller square (2) in the lower corner (Figure 11-3). The smaller square is one-ninth of the area of the larger square. Using random fields in which the RBCs are evenly distributed, the reticulocytes found in both the large and small squares are quantitated while the number of RBCs counted in the small square reaches at least 200.

The percentage of reticulocytes is determined using the following formula:

$$\% \text{ Reticulocytes} = \frac{\text{\# Reticulocytes in squares 1 and 2} \times 100}{\text{\# RBCs in square 2} \qquad \times 9}$$

The factor of 9 is used in the denominator because the ratio of the area in which the RBCs are counted to the total square is 1:9.

PROBLEMS

A reticulocyte count was performed on a patient using the Miller disc method. A total of 28 reticulocytes were counted, along with 222 RBCs. What is the patient's reticulocyte count?

Using the formula for calculating reticulocytes using the Miller disc, and substituting into it the data from the problem, the following equation is derived:

$$\% \text{ Reticulocytes} = \frac{\text{\# Reticulocytes in squares 1 and 2 (28)} \times 100}{\text{\# RBCs in square 2 (222)} \qquad \times 9}$$

$$= \frac{28}{1998} \times 100$$

$$= 0.014 \times 100$$

$$= 1.4\%$$

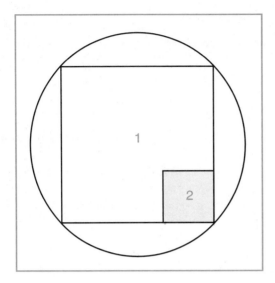

FIGURE 11-3 Miller disc.

A reticulocyte count was performed on a patient using the Miller disc method. A total of 17 reticulocytes were counted, along with 205 RBCs. What is the patient's reticulocyte count?

Using the formula for calculating reticulocytes using the Miller disc, and substituting into it the data from the problem, the following equation is derived:

$$\% \text{ Reticulocytes} = \frac{\text{\# Reticulocytes in squares 1 and 2 (17)} \times 100}{\text{\# RBCs in square 2 (205)} \times 9}$$

$$= \frac{17}{1845} \times 100$$

$$= 0.009 \times 100$$

$$= 0.9\%$$

Rh Incompatibility

Approximately 15% of the population lacks the RBC antigen D and is therefore considered to be Rh negative. An Rh negative individual does not naturally have circulating antibodies to the D antigen. Rh negative mothers who are carrying Rh positive fetuses may run the risk of antibody production. Fetal-maternal bleeds can occur with any pregnancy, and maternal and fetal blood may be mixed at delivery. In most cases, an Rh negative mother with an Rh positive fetus will not become sensitized to the Rh factor unless a fetal-maternal bleed occurs. In the mid-1960s, it was discovered that if nonsensitized Rh negative individuals received intramuscular doses of Rh immune globulin, their immune systems failed to produce D antibodies even after exposure to the D antigen. This finding ultimately led to the current immunization of Rh negative pregnant women during and immediately after delivery with Rh immune globulin (RhIG).

Determining the Quantity of RhIG to Administer

It has been estimated that the average fetal-maternal bleed contains approximately 30 mL of whole blood or 15 mL of packed RBCs. RhIG is formulated to contain 300 μg of RhIG, which is sufficient to protect against an average bleed. One unit of RhIG is generally sufficient to protect an Rh negative pregnant woman during pregnancy, and a second dose is administered within 72 hours of delivery. However, there may be cases of increased fetal-maternal bleeding. In these cases, the number of RhIG units must be calculated to prevent antibody formation. The Kleihauer-Betke acid elution test is performed, and the percentage of fetal cells is determined. Some laboratories utilize the more exact flow cytometry method to quantitate fetal cells. The number of units or vials of RhIG to be administered is calculated by the following formula:

$$\text{Vials of RhIG} = \frac{\% \text{ fetal cells} \times 50}{30}$$

where

    % fetal cells = number of fetal cells per 1000 maternal cells
              50 = factor used to account for average maternal blood volume
              30 = average quantity of fetal-maternal bleed (mL)

In order to err on the side of caution, the result is rounded to the nearest whole number, and an additional unit is added.

PROBLEMS

A woman was rushed into the emergency room hemorrhaging from a miscarriage. Her blood type was B Rh negative, and the father was A positive. A Kleihaeur-Betke acid elution test determined the percentage of fetal cells in the mother's circulation to be 2.8%. How many units of RhIG should the woman be given to prevent the formation of D antibodies?

The formula to determine the units of RhIG is:

$$\text{Vials of RhIG} = \frac{\% \text{ fetal cells} \times 50}{30}$$

where

    % fetal cells = number of fetal cells per 1000 maternal cells
              50 = factor used to account for average maternal blood volume
              30 = average quantity of fetal-maternal bleed (mL)

Substituting into the formula the data from the problem:

$$\text{Vials of RhIG} = \frac{2.8\% \times 50}{30}$$

$$= 4.7$$

The amount calculated, 4.7, is rounded to 5.0, and an additional vial is added to err on the side of safety. Therefore, the woman would receive six vials of RhIG.

A woman who was 12 weeks pregnant arrived at her gynecologist's office with profuse uterine bleeding. Her blood type was A Rh negative, and the father was O positive. A Kleihaeur-Betke acid elution test determined the percentage of fetal cells in the mother's circulation to be 1.7%. How many units of RhIG should the woman be given to prevent the formation of D antibodies?

Using the formula to determine the units of RhIG results in the following equation:

$$\text{Vials of RhIG} = \frac{1.7\% \times 50}{30}$$

$$= 2.8$$

The amount calculated, 2.8, is rounded to 3.0, and an additional vial is added to err on the side of safety. Therefore, the woman would receive four vials of RhIG.

EXAMPLE PROBLEMS

This section is designed to be useful to both the student and the health care practitioner. Students can use the example problems in order to master the material. The health care practitioner can use these problems as templates for solving laboratory calculations. Find an example problem similar to the problem that you need to solve and substitute into the equation the numbers appropriate to your calculation.

1. **Q Calculate the MCV of a sample if the hematocrit is 35% and the RBC count is 4.0 (million per μL).**

    A The MCV is calculated from the following formula:

    $$\text{MCV (fL)} = \frac{\text{Hct} \times 10}{\text{RBC count}}$$

    Substituting into the formula the data from the problem yields:

    $$\text{MCV (fL)} = \frac{35 \times 10}{4}$$

    $$= 87.5 \text{ fL.}$$

2. **Q Calculate the MCV of a sample with a hematocrit of 42% and an RBC count of 5.2 (million per μL).**

    A Using the formula for MCV, the following equation is derived:

    $$\text{MCV (fL)} = \frac{42\% \times 10}{5.2}$$

    $$= 81 \text{ fL.}$$

3. **Q** **Calculate the MCH of a sample with a hemoglobin concentration of 13 g/dL and an RBC count of 3.7 (millions per μL).**

   A The MCH is calculated by the following formula:

   $$\text{MCH (pg)} = \frac{\text{Hemoglobin (g/dL)} \times 10}{\text{RBC count}}$$

   $$= \frac{13 \times 10}{3.7}$$

   $$= 35 \text{ pg.}$$

4. **Q** **Calculate the MCH of a sample with a hemoglobin concentration of 16 g/dL and an RBC count of 4.8 (millions per μL).**

   A Using the formula:

   $$\text{MCH (pg)} = \frac{16 \text{ g/dL} \times 10}{4.8}$$

   $$= 33 \text{ pg.}$$

5. **Q** **Calculate the MCHC of a sample with a hemoglobin concentration of 10 g/dL and a hematocrit of 30%.**

   A The MCHC is calculated by the following formula:

   $$\text{MCHC (\%)} = \frac{\text{Hb (g/dL)} \times 100}{\text{Hematocrit (\%)}}$$

   Substituting into the formula the data from the problem:

   $$\text{MCHC (\%)} = \frac{10 \times 100}{30\%}$$

   $$= 33\%.$$

6. **Q** **A WBC count was performed on a 1/20 dilution using the four corner squares of the hemacytometer. The number of WBCs counted was 210. What is the total number of WBCs?**

   A Since the WBC count was performed using the standard dilution and counting technique, the total WBC count is 210 × 50 or 10,500/ mm³.

7. **Q** **A manual WBC count was performed on a sample from a patient with a history of low WBC counts. A 1/10 dilution was performed, and the WBCs found in all nine squares were counted—a total of 66 WBCs. What is the patient's total WBC count?**

   A The factor method cannot be used to calculate this patient's WBC count because the standard parameters were not used. The formula for calculating cells/mm³ is as follows:

   $$\text{\# Cells/mm}^3 = \frac{\text{\# cells counted} \times \text{depth factor} \times \text{dilution factor}}{\text{Area counted}}$$

In this case, the number of cells counted is 66, the depth factor is still 10, the dilution factor is 10, not 20, and the total area counted is nine, not four. Therefore, by substituting into the formula the known data, the total WBC count can be calculated:

$$WBCs/mm^3 = \frac{66 \times 10 \times 10}{9}$$

$$= 733.$$

8. **Q** **A WBC count was performed using a hemacytometer and a ¹/₂₀ dilution. A total of 157 WBCs were counted in the four large corner squares of the hemacytometer. Using the factor method, what is the total WBC count?**

A In the mathematical formula used to calculate the factor:

Factor = 1/area × depth factor × dilution factor

Area counted = number of large squares counted

Depth factor = reciprocal of depth [1/(¹/₁₀)] = 10

Dilution factor = reciprocal of dilution = [1/(¹/₂₀)] = 20

Therefore, the factor is:

$$\frac{1}{4} \times 10 \times 20 = 50.$$

Therefore, the number of cells counted, 157, times the factor, 50, is equal to the total WBC count: 157 × 50 = 7850/mm³.

> **Note** The factor method can be used to count WBCs *only* if the dilution performed is ¹/₂₀ and all WBCs in the four large corner squares are counted.

9. **Q** **A WBC count was performed using a ¹/₂₀ dilution. All WBCs in the four large corner squares of the hemacytometer were counted, resulting in a count of 314 WBCs. What is the total WBC count?**

A Because the dilution performed was ¹/₂₀ and all WBCs in the four large corner squares of the hemacytometer were counted, the factor method can be used. The total WBC count is equal to the factor of 50 multiplied by the number of WBCs counted. Therefore, the total WBC count is 15,700/mm³ or, equivalently, $15,700 \times 10^9$/L.

10. **Q** **A manual RBC count was performed on a sample that was diluted ¹/₂₀₀. Within the 80 small squares in the center square, 484 RBCs were counted. What is the total RBC count in terms of 10^6/mm³?**

A The factor method can also be used to count RBCs. In the factor method:

$$\text{Factor} = 1/\text{area} \times \text{depth factor} \times \text{dilution factor}$$
$$\text{Area counted} = \text{area of small squares counted}$$
$$\text{Depth factor} = \text{reciprocal of depth } [1/(^1/_{10})] = 10$$
$$\text{Dilution factor} = \text{reciprocal of dilution} = [1/(^1/_{200})] = 200$$

Therefore, the factor is:

$$\frac{1}{0.2} \times 10 \times 200 = 10{,}000.$$

To determine the total RBC count, multiply the number of cells counted, 484, by the factor of 10,000; $484 \times 10{,}000 = 4{,}840{,}000/\text{mm}^3$ or $4.84 \times 10^6/\text{mm}^3$.

11. **Q** **An RBC count is performed following the standard dilution and counting technique. The number of RBCs counted is 495. What is the total RBC count?**

A The factor of 10,000 may be used to solve this problem since standard parameters were used. Therefore, the total RBC count/mm³ is 10,000 $\times 495 = 4{,}950{,}000/\text{mm}^3$ or $4.95 \times 10^6/\text{mm}^3$.

12. **Q** **An RBC count was performed using a $^1/_{100}$ dilution on a sample from a patient with severe anemia. A total of 194 RBCs were counted within the 80 small squares found in the center square of the hemacytometer. What is the total RBC count?**

A The factor method cannot be used to solve this problem because a $^1/_{100}$ dilution was performed. Instead, the following formula is used:

$$\# \text{ Cells/mm}^3 = \frac{\# \text{ Cells counted} \times \text{depth factor} \times \text{dilution factor}}{\text{Area counted}}$$

In this case, the number of cells counted is 194, the depth factor remains the same, 10, the dilution factor is 100, and the area counted is 0.2. Substituting into the equation the known values leads to the following equation:

$$\# \text{ RBCs/mm}^3 = \frac{94 \times 10 \times 100}{0.2}$$
$$= 970{,}000 \quad \text{or} \quad 9.7 \times 10^5/\text{mm}^3.$$

13. **Q** **A platelet count was performed using a $^1/_{100}$ dilution, and all platelets found in the 400 smallest squares of the central square in the hemacytometer were counted—a total of 275 platelets. What is the platelet count?**

A A factor can also be used to quantify platelets. However, a $^1/_{100}$ dilution must be performed, and all platelets found in the 25 smallest squares within the central square must be counted. Each of the 25 squares is further divided into 16 squares. Therefore, the total number of squares counted is 400 (16 × 25). In the formula used to derive the factor for platelets:

$$\text{Factor} = 1/\text{area} \times \text{depth factor} \times \text{dilution factor}$$
$$\text{Area counted} = \text{area of small squares counted}$$
$$(0.04 \times 25 = 1 \text{ mm}^2)$$
$$\text{Depth factor} = \text{reciprocal of depth } [1/(^1/_{10})] = 10$$
$$\text{Dilution factor} = \text{reciprocal of dilution} = [1/(^1/_{100})] = 100$$

Therefore, the factor is:

$$\frac{1}{1.0} \times 10 \times 100 = 1{,}000.$$

The number of platelets counted is multiplied by the factor to calculate the total platelet count: 275 × 1000 = 275,000/mm³.

14. **Q** **A platelet count was performed using a ¹/₁₀₀ dilution, and 124 platelets were counted in the platelet counting area of the hemacytometer. What is the total platelet count?**

A The factor method can be used for this problem because standard parameters were used. The number of platelets counted, 124, multiplied by the factor of 1000 is equal to a platelet count of 124,000/mm³.

15. **Q** **A platelet count was performed on a chemotherapy patient. A ¹/₅₀ dilution was used, and all 400 small squares within the central square were counted, for a total number of 16 platelets. What is the total platelet count?**

A The factor method cannot be used to solve this problem because a ¹/₅₀ dilution, not a ¹/₁₀₀ dilution, was performed. Instead, use the following formula:

$$\text{Cells/mm}^3 = \frac{\text{\# Cells counted} \times \text{depth factor} \times \text{dilution factor}}{\text{Area counted}}$$
$$= \frac{16 \times 10 \times 50}{1 \text{ mm}^2}$$
$$= 8000/\text{mm}^3.$$

16. **Q** **A reticulocyte count was performed, and 27 reticulocytes were counted per 1000 RBCs. What is the reticulocyte percentage?**

A The formula to calculate reticulocytes is:

$$\frac{\text{\# Reticulocytes counted per 1000 erythrocytes}}{1000} \times 100$$

Using the formula and substituting the data from the problem:

$$\frac{27}{1000} \times 100 = 2.7\%.$$

Therefore, the reticulocyte count is 2.7%.

17. **Q** **A reticulocyte count is performed, and 13 reticulocytes are found among 1000 mature RBCs. What is the reticulocyte percentage?**

A Using the formula for reticulocytes:

$$\frac{24}{1000} \times 100 = 1.3\%.$$

Therefore, the reticulocyte percentage is 1.3%.

18. **Q** **A reticulocyte count was performed using the Miller disc method. A total of 26 reticulocytes were counted, along with 245 RBCs. What is the patient's reticulocyte count?**

A The Miller disc is a calibrated glass insert for the eyepiece lens of the microscope. The glass insert has a large center square (square 1 in Figure 11-3) within which is a smaller square (square 2 in Figure 11-3) in the lower corner. The reticulocytes within both the large and small squares are counted until the number of RBCs counted only in the small corner square (square 2) reaches at least 200. The following formula is used to determine the percentage of reticulocytes with a Miller disc:

$$\frac{\text{\# Reticulocytes in squares 1 and 2}}{\text{(\# RBCs in square 2)(9)}} \times 100$$

Substituting into the equation the values from the problem:

$$\frac{\text{\# Reticulocytes in small and large squares (26)}}{\text{\# RBCs in square 2 (245)} \times 9} \times 100$$

$$\% \text{ Reticulocytes} = \frac{26}{2205} \times 100$$

$$= 0.012 \times 100$$

$$= 1.2\%.$$

19. **Q** **A reticulocyte count was performed using the Miller disc method, and 53 reticulocytes were counted among 230 RBCs. What is the reticulocyte percentage?**

A Using the formula for the Miller disc method, the following equation is derived:

$$\frac{\text{\# Reticulocytes in small and large squares (53)}}{\text{\# RBCs in square 2(230)} \times 9} \times 100$$

$$\% \text{ Reticulocytes} = \frac{53}{2070} \times 100$$

$$= 0.026 \times 100$$

$$= 2.6\%.$$

20. **Q** **A pregnant woman presented with premature rupture of membranes. The woman's blood type was group AB Rh negative, and**

the father was group O Rh positive. A Kleihaeur-Betke acid elution test determined the percentage of fetal cells in the mother's circulation to be 3.7%. How many vials of RhIG should the woman be given to prevent the formation of D antibodies?

A It is estimated that the average fetal-maternal bleed contains approximately 30 mL of whole blood or 15 mL of packed RBCs. Each vial of RhIG is formulated to contain 300 µg of immune globulin that is sufficient to protect against an average bleed. When a pregnant woman experiences increased bleeding, the following formula is used to determine the number of vials of RhIG necessary to prevent antibody formation.

$$\text{Vials of RhIG} = \frac{\% \text{ Fetal cells} \times 50}{30}$$

where:

% fetal cells = number of fetal cells per 1000 maternal cells

50 = factor used to account for average maternal blood volume

30 = average quantity of fetal-maternal bleed

Substituting into the formula the data from the problem:

$$\text{Vials of RhIG} = \frac{3.7\% \times 50}{30}$$

$$= 6.2.$$

The amount calculated, 6.2, is rounded to 6.0, and an additional vial is added to err on the side of safety. Therefore, the woman would receive seven vials of RhIG.

21. **Q** An Rh negative pregnant woman carrying an Rh positive fetus was a passenger in an automobile that crashed. The woman received blunt trauma to the lower abdomen. An ultrasound exam revealed damage to the placenta. The percentage of fetal cells within the woman's circulation was calculated by the Kleihaeur-Betke acid elution test to be 2.5%. How many vials of RhIG should the woman receive to prevent the formation of D antibodies?

A Substituting into the formula used to determine the number of vials of RhIG to administer the data from the problem, the following equation is derived:

$$\text{Vials of RhIG} = \frac{2.5\% \text{ fetal cells} \times 50}{30}$$

$$= 4.2.$$

Therefore, five vials of RhIG will be administered to the patient.

Solve the following practice problems to further master the material. All answers and explanations to some problems can be found in a separate section at the back of the book.

Calculate the MCV given the following information:
  1. Hematocrit = 21%, RBC count   = 3.2 (million per µL)
  2. Hematocrit = 45%, RBC count   = 4.5 (million per µL)
  3. Hematocrit = 33%, RBC count   = 2.7 (million per µL)

Calculate the MCH given the following information:
  4. Hemoglobin = 10 g/dL, RBC count = 3.0 (million per µL)
  5. Hemoglobin = 18 g/dL, RBC count = 3.7 (million per µL)
  6. Hemoglobin = 14 g/dL, RBC count = 3.3 (million per µL)

Calculate the MCHC given the following information:
  7. Hemoglobin = 16 g/dL, hematocrit = 36%
  8. Hemoglobin = 5 g/dL, hematocrit = 15%
  9. Hemoglobin = 15 g/dL, hematocrit = 45%

For the following WBC counts performed on a $\frac{1}{20}$ dilution and counting all WBCs in the four large corner squares of the hemacytometer, use the factor method to calculate the WBC count/mm^3.
10. 74 WBCs counted
11. 145 WBCs counted
12. 92 WBCs counted

For the following RBC counts performed on a $\frac{1}{200}$ dilution and counting all RBCs within the five squares used within the center square of the hemacytometer, use the factor method to calculate the RBC count/mm^3.
13. 487 RBCs counted
14. 269 RBCs counted
15. 615 RBCs counted

For the following platelet counts performed on a $\frac{1}{100}$ dilution and counting all platelets within the center square of the hemacytometer, use the factor method to calculate the platelet count/mm^3.
16. 222 platelets counted
17. 68 platelets counted
18. 142 platelets counted

Calculate the following cell counts without using the factor method:
19. WBC count: $1/10$ dilution performed, 78 WBCs counted in four corner squares
20. WBC count: $1/20$ dilution performed, 120 WBCs counted in eight large squares
21. RBC count: $1/100$ dilution performed, 318 RBCs counted in four corner squares and the middle square within the center square
22. RBC count: $1/100$ dilution performed, 236 RBCs counted in four corner squares and the middle square within the center square
23. Platelet count: $1/50$ dilution, 197 platelets counted within the large center square
24. Platelet count: $1/100$ dilution, 66 platelets counted in the four large corner squares usually used for WBC counts

Calculate the percentage of reticulocytes given the following data:
25. 46 reticulocytes counted per 1000 RBCs
26. 18 reticulocytes counted per 1000 RBCs
27. 65 reticulocytes counted in the large and small squares of the Miller disc, and 208 RBCs counted in square 2 of the Miller disc
28. 40 reticulocytes counted in the large and small squares of the Miller disc, and 203 RBCs counted in square 2 of the Miller disc

Determine the number of vials of RhIG necessary to prevent D antibody formation in the following pregnant women:
29. Percentage of fetal cells in maternal circulation = 2.9%.
30. Percentage of fetal cells in maternal circulation = 1.2%.

CHAPTER 12

Microbiology Laboratory

INTRODUCTION

Colony Counts

The colony count determines the amount of bacteria present in a sample. It is often used in the microbiology laboratory to determine the amount of bacteria present in a urine sample. Urine is a sterile fluid formed by the kidney and stored in the bladder until voided. As urine passes from the bladder into the urethra, it may become contaminated with the normal flora found in the urethra. Bacteria on the skin in the genital area may also contaminate the urine specimen. The total amount of bacteria present due to contamination is less than 10,000 organisms per milliliter of urine or less than 10,000 (10^3) colony-forming units (CFU). Urinary tract infections are caused primarily by single strains of bacteria. Infections caused by more than one strain are not very common. If three strains of organisms are detected, contamination of the specimen has most likely occurred. The most common organism responsible for urinary tract infections is *Escherichia coli,* a gram-negative rod. When a physician suspects that a patient has a urinary tract infection, a clean-catch urine sample is collected by the patient. When the concentration of organisms is greater than 100,000 per milliliter (10^5 CFU), a urinary tract infection is indicated. If a urine sample is to be used for both microbiological studies and urinalysis, the microbiological studies are performed first to avoid contamination of the sample with reagent strips, pipettes, and so on. A colony count is performed by first using a calibrated loop to inoculate a culture plate. Two different calibrated loops can be used; one loop holds 0.01 mL of sample, and the other loop holds 0.001 mL.

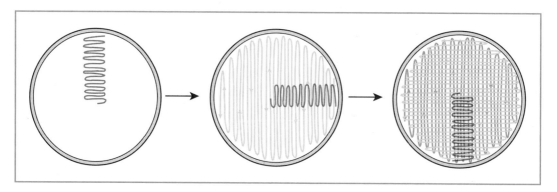

The urine is streaked first with a primary streak down the middle of the plate. Then the plate is turned 90 degrees and streaked across the primary streak the length of the plate. Finally, the plate is again turned 90 degrees (or 180 degrees from the original orientation) and streaked across the secondary streaks. In this manner, the entire plate is streaked with urine, and any organisms can be isolated. The plate is incubated aerobically at 37°C for 24 hours, and the number of colonies or CFU is counted. Each CFU represents a single organism from the original sample. The total number of CFU is calculated by multiplying the number of colonies by the dilution factor of the calibrated loop. If a 0.01 calibrated loop is used, the number of colonies counted is multiplied by 100. If a 0.001 calibrated loop is used, the number of colonies counted is multiplied by 1000. In this manner, the total number of CFU per milliliter of urine can be determined. Clean-catch urine specimens that contain less than 10^3 CFU of bacteria do not indicate a urinary tract infection. Clean-catch urine specimens that contain between 10^3 and 10^5 CFU indicate a possible infection. When a possible infection is indicated, the organism is identified and antibiotic susceptibility testing is performed. Clean-catch urine specimens that contain more than 10^5 CFU indicate probable infection. As with a possible infection, the organism is identified and antibiotic susceptibility testing is performed.

Urine may also be collected from an indwelling catheter. Patients with indwelling catheters are at high risk of acquiring urinary tract infections, so sterile technique should be carefully followed. Urine is never collected for culture from the collection bag. Significant bacteriuria is indicated if more than 10^5 CFU are counted.

Urine may also be collected by suprapubic aspiration. In this surgical procedure, urine is taken directly from the bladder and cultured. Any CFU detected should be reported, the organism identified, and antibiotic susceptibility testing performed.

PROBLEMS

A clean-catch urine specimen is obtained from a 32-year-old woman with a possible urinary tract infection. The urine is cultured using a 0.01 mL calibrated loop. After appropriate incubation, 215 colonies are counted. What is the patient's CFU/mL count, and does it indicate a urinary tract infection?

A 0.01 mL calibrated loop was used to inoculate this urine specimen. Therefore, the number of colonies, 215, is multiplied by the dilution factor of 100, yielding 21,500 CFU/mL.

A CFU count of at least 10^5 is necessary to indicate probable infection. The patient's CFU/mL count was 2.2×10^4, indicating possible, but not probable, infection.

A clean-catch urine specimen is obtained from a 25-year-old woman with a possible urinary tract infection. The urine is cultured using a 0.01 mL calibrated loop. After appropriate incubation, 1382 colonies are counted. What is the patient's CFU/mL count, and does it indicate a urinary tract infection?

A 0.01 mL calibrated loop was used to inoculate this urine specimen. Therefore, the number of colonies, 1382, is multiplied by the dilution factor of 100, yielding 138,200 CFU/mL.

A CFU count of at least 10^5 is necessary to indicate probable infection. The patient's CFU/mL count was 1.38×10^5, indicating probable infection.

A urine specimen obtained by catheter from an 8-month-old girl is cultured for possible infection using a 0.001 mL calibrated loop. Following standard laboratory protocol, 110 organisms are counted. What is the baby's CFU/mL count, and does it indicate an infection?

Since a 0.001 mL calibrated loop was used to inoculate the urine specimen, the number of colonies counted, 110, is multiplied by 1000, yielding 1.1×10^5 CFU/mL. This number of organisms indicates a probable infection.

A clean-catch urine specimen is obtained from a 2-year-old boy with a possible urinary tract infection. The urine is cultured using a 0.001 mL calibrated loop. After appropriate incubation, 85 colonies are counted. What is the patient's CFU/mL count, and does it indicate a urinary tract infection?

A 0.001 mL calibrated loop was used to inoculate this urine. Therefore, the number of colonies, 85, is multiplied by the dilution factor of 1000, yielding 85,000 CFU/mL.

A CFU count of at least 10^5 is necessary to indicate probable infection. The patient's CFU/mL count was 8.5×10^4, indicating possible, but not probable, infection.

Antimicrobial Susceptibility Testing

Once an organism is identified as a possible pathogen, the microbiology laboratory must identify the possible antimicrobial(s) that can kill or inhibit the growth of the organism. An organism that is inhibited completely by a particular antimicrobial is said to be *susceptible* to that antimicrobial. If the organism continues to grow when exposed to the antimicrobial, the organism is considered to be *resistant* to that antimicrobial. The dose of antimicrobial to be given to the patient should be the lowest possible dose that will inhibit or kill the organism. This dose is termed the *minimum inhibitory concentration (MIC)* and is measured in micrograms per milliliter (µg/mL). The MIC for a particular antimicrobial can be determined in either broth or agar. The broth test can be performed either by tube (macrotube) or by microtiter plate (microtube). There are automated instruments that are capable of reading the microtiter MIC plates.

To perform a macrotube broth MIC test, a standard suspension of the test organism is first prepared. Four or five colonies are placed in a suitable broth (usually Mueller-Hinton [MH] or tryptic soy broth [TSB]) and vortexed until the turbidity of the broth is that of a 0.5 McFarland standard suspension. McFarland standard suspensions are solutions of varying concentrations of barium sulfate and sulfuric acid. By forming increasingly turbid samples, the standards represent increasing numbers of bacteria in suspension. A 0.5 McFarland standard suspension represents a bacterial suspension containing 10^8 CFU/mL of organism. Appendix A contains information on the preparation of the 0.5 McFarland standard suspension. Typically, the broth inoculum is diluted $^1/_{100}$ to yield a concentration of 10^6 CFU/mL prior to inoculation into the antibiotic. The standard MIC dilutional scheme will result in a final diluted inoculum concentration in each tube of 5×10^5 CFU/mL.

To begin the dilutional scheme, 1 mL of MH broth is added to 12 sterile test tubes. One of the test tubes is kept aside, as it will be the control. The control test tube can be labeled tube 13. Next, 2 mL of the stock antimicrobial is placed in a test tube, which is labeled tube 1. Then, a twofold serial dilution using 1 mL

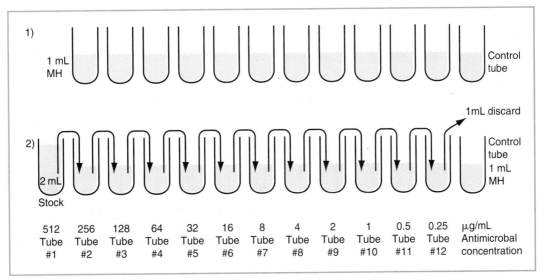

FIGURE 12-1 Macrobroth MIC dilutional scheme (partial). (From Doucette, L. J. [1997]. *Mathematics for the Clinical Laboratory* [p. 247]. Philadelphia: W.B. Saunders Company.)

of the stock antimicrobial, is performed on the 11 remaining tubes (labeled 2–12). For the last tube (tube 12), after the tube is mixed, 1 mL is discarded so that the total volume is still 1 mL. Figure 12-1 is a schematic of a procedure using ampicillin as the antimicrobial to be tested up to this point.

Note that the antimicrobial is diluted serially in this dilutional scheme. In the next step, the antimicrobial will be further diluted. Next, 1 mL of the test organism at a concentration of 1×10^6 CFU/mL is added to each tube, including control tube 13. When 1 mL is added to the 1 mL already in the tube, the antimicrobial and the test organism are diluted by one-half. Therefore, in the 12 tubes, the concentration of the test organism is 5×10^5 CFU/mL (one-half of 1×10^6), and the concentration of the antimicrobial ranges from 256 to 0.125 μg/mL, as demonstrated in Figure 12-2.

The 13 tubes are incubated overnight at 35°C. They are then checked for the presence of turbidity, which represents growth of the organism in the antimicrobial. The MIC is the lowest concentration of antimicrobial in which there is no growth.

PROBLEM

A wound culture containing *Staphylococcus* aureus was obtained from a 52-year-old diabetic woman. The physician wishes the MIC for the antimicrobial vancomycin to be determined. The concentration of the stock antimicrobial in MH broth is 512 μg/mL. Using 12 tubes, a twofold serial dilution of 1 mL of the stock antimicrobial into 1 mL of MH broth is performed.

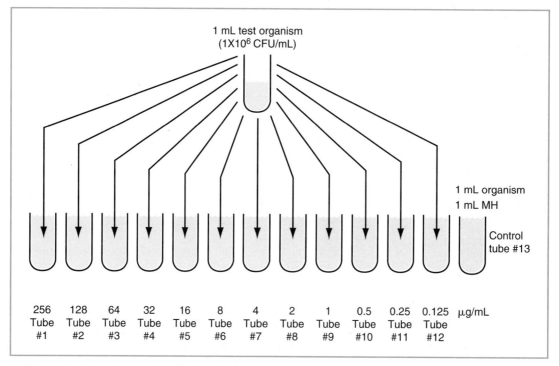

FIGURE 12-2　Macrobroth MIC dilutional scheme (completed). (From Doucette, L. J. [1997]. *Mathematics for the Clinical Laboratory* [p. 248]. Philadelphia: W.B. Saunders Company.)

What is the concentration of antimicrobial in tube 4?

The first tube in the series has an antimicrobial concentration of 256 µg/mL, the second tube's concentration is 128 µg/mL, the third tube's concentration is 64 µg/mL, and the fourth tube's concentration is 32 µg/mL.

EXAMPLE PROBLEMS

This section is designed to be useful to both the student and the health care practitioner. Students can use the example problems in order to master the material. The health care practitioner can use these problems as templates for performing laboratory calculations. Find an example problem similar to the problem that you need to solve and substitute into the equation the numbers appropriate to your calculation.

1. **Q** **A urine specimen was obtained for a culture and sensitivity test. A 0.01 calibrated loop was used to streak the plate. After appropriate incubation, 345 CFU were counted. Does this indicate a urinary tract infection?**

   A Since a 0.01 mL calibrated loop was used to inoculate the culture plate, the number of CFU found on the plate is multiplied by the dilution factor of 100. In this problem, there are 34,500 CFU/mL. The patient's CFU count indicates a possible infection. However, a count of at least 10^5 CFU/mL is necessary to indicate a probable urinary tract infection.

2. **Q** **A urine specimen was cultured using a 0.001 calibrated loop, and 97 CFU were counted after appropriate incubation. Does this indicate a urinary tract infection?**

   A When a 0.001 calibrated loop is used to inoculate a urine specimen, the number of colonies counted is multiplied by the dilution factor of 1000. In this case, there are 97,000 CFU/mL, which indicates a probable urinary tract infection.

3. **Q** **A urine specimen was cultured using a 0.001 calibrated loop, and 8 CFU were cultured after appropriate incubation. Does this indicate a urinary tract infection?**

   A The number of colonies, 8, is multiplied by the dilution factor, 1000, to yield a total of 8000 CFU/mL for this specimen. This value indicates contamination, but not a probable or possible urinary tract infection.

4. **Q** **What is the MIC?**

   A The MIC is the minimum inhibitory concentration of an antimicrobial. MIC tests are used to assess the dosage of antimicrobial necessary to inhibit the growth of organisms.

5. **Q** **How is an MIC test performed?**

   A MIC tests can be performed on broth or agar, in tubes (macro method), or on microtiter plates (micro method). The organisms are adjusted in broth to a density of a McFarland 0.5 standard suspension. In the macrotube method, an equal amount of MH broth is added to 12 tubes. Then, a serial dilution of the antimicrobial to be tested is performed in the tubes. An equal amount of the test organism is then added to each tube, and the tubes are incubated overnight. The MIC is the lowest concentration in which there is no visual growth of the organism.

PRACTICE PROBLEMS

Solve the following problems to further master the material. All answers and explanations to some problems can be found in a separate section at the back of the book.

1. If 1355 CFU were counted on a urine culture that was inoculated with a 0.01 mL calibrated loop, what is the concentration of CFU/mL?
2. If 169 CFU were counted on a urine culture that was inoculated with a 0.01 calibrated loop, what is the concentration of CFU/mL?
3. If 134 CFU were counted on a urine culture that was inoculated with a 0.001 mL calibrated loop, what is the concentration of CFU/mL?
4. If 7 CFU were counted on a urine culture that was inoculated with a 0.001 calibrated loop, what is the concentration of CFU/mL?
5. At what concentration of bacteria is a urinary tract infection possible if the urine sample was a clean-catch sample?
6. At what concentration of bacteria is a urinary tract infection probable if the urine sample was a clean-catch sample?
7. In a macrobroth MIC, which tube has a *final* antibiotic concentration of 0.5 µg/mL?

BIBLIOGRAPHY

Baron, E., Peterson, L., and Finegold, S. *Bailey & Scott's Diagnostic Microbiology*, 9th ed. Mosby, St. Louis, 1994.

National Committee for Clinical Laboratory Standards. *Methods for Dilution Antimicrobial Susceptibility Tests for Bacteria That Grow Aerobically*, 2nd ed., M7-A2. Villanova, PA, 1990.

Rowland, S., Walsh, S., Teel, L., and Carnahan, A. *Pathogenic and Clinical Microbiology: A Laboratory Manual*. Little, Brown and Company, Boston, 1994.

CHAPTER 13

Quality Assurance in the Clinical Laboratory: Basic Statistical Concepts

INTRODUCTION

Basic Statistical Concepts

Laboratory tests should be accurate and precise, and statistical analysis of data is one tool that can help us achieve this goal. Some basic statistical terms must be learned first to better understand the analysis of data.

Mean

The mean is the *average* of a group of numbers. In statistical analysis its symbol is $\overline{X}$, an X with a bar over it. We sometimes use the mean value to perform other statistical tests on the group. The mean is one indicator of *central tendency*, the distribution of data around a central value.

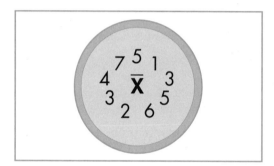

PROBLEMS

An administrator for a small rural hospital asked, "What is the mean for the average length of stay for postoperative patients during a representative 1 week period?"

There were 15 patients who stayed for various amounts of time. Their length of stay in minutes is as follows:

Patient	Length of Stay
1	325
2	130
3	65
4	95
5	128
6	42
7	140
8	35
9	240
10	45

11	90
12	55
13	120
14	150
15	38

To calculate the mean, first add the 15 length-of-stay values:

$$325 + 130 + 65 + 95 + 128 + 42 + 140 + 35 + 240 + 45 + 90 + 55 + 120 + 150 + 38 = 1698$$

Next, divide the sum by the total number of lengths of stay, in this case 15. The total quantity in a set of numbers is referred to as *n*.

$$\frac{1698}{n \text{ or } 15} = 113$$

Therefore, the mean value for this group of length-of-stay values is 113 minutes.

A medical laboratory technician was establishing the mean for a new lot number of quality control material to be used for a cholesterol test. He analyzed the material 20 times to generate sufficient data for his calculations. Given the values for the 20 cholesterol results that were obtained, calculate the mean cholesterol value for this quality control material.

Quality control results: 205, 210, 206, 198, 199, 201, 207, 212, 203, 200, 205, 207, 202, 211, 209, 213, 200, 200, 204, 210

The mean is determined by the following equation:

$$\frac{\text{Sum of QC results}}{n \text{ or } 20}$$

The mean for the quality control material is 205, determined by the sum, 4102, divided by the *n* value of 20.

Median

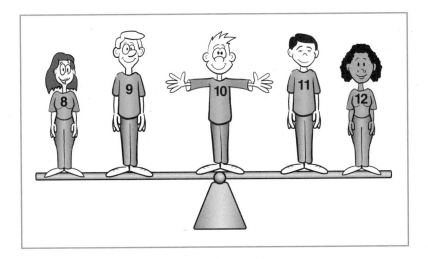

Another indicator of central tendency is the *median,* the central number in a group of numbers arranged in sequential order. That is, just as many numbers are above the median value as are below it. The median value may or may not be the same as the mean value.

PROBLEMS

Using the following group of numbers, find the median value.

4, 6, 7, 2, 8, 3, 6, 5, 1

To find the median value, first rank the numbers from lowest to highest in value.

Lowest 1
       2
       3
       4
       5
       6
       6
       7
Highest 8

Note that the total number of values (nine) in this set of values is an odd number. To determine the median of a set of values that contains an odd number of values, first add 1 to the total number of values, in this case nine. Divide the total number of values (plus one) by 2.

In this example, there are nine values.

$$9 + 1 = 10$$
$$\frac{10}{2} = 5$$

Next, go down the list to the fifth number on the list, which is 5. This number is the median value for this group of numbers.

> **Note** This method of determining the median is used more commonly when the group of numbers is large. If the group of numbers is small, simply ranking the numbers in ascending order and finding the middle number in the group is all that is necessary to determine the median value.

Lowest 1
       2
       3
       4
       5 Median

6
6
7
Highest 8

Note that there is an equal number of values above and below the median value.

Given the following set of numbers, determine the median number.

31, 35, 37, 31, 30, 34, 36

Rank the numbers in ascending order:

30
31
31
34
35
36
37

The median number is the middle number, 34.

In the previous example, the group consisted of seven values, an odd number. If the group consists of an even number of values, the median must be calculated slightly differently. Below are a group of numbers. What is the median value?

21, 24, 19, 20, 22, 23, 21, 25

The first step is to arrange the numbers in order from lowest to highest value.

Lowest 19
20
21
21
22
23
24
Highest 25

Next, divide the total numbers in this group by 2. There are eight numbers in this group.

$$\frac{8}{2} = 4$$

Next, add 1 to this value:

$$4 + 1 = 5$$

The median in this group of numbers is found to be the average of the fourth and fifth numbers in this group.

Lowest 19
      20
      21
      21 fourth number; average of the fourth and fifth numbers is 21.5
      22 fifth number
      23
      24
Highest 25

The median for this group of numbers is 21.5. Note that there is an equal number of values above and below the median value.

PROBLEM

Determine the median value for the following group of numbers:

   3, 5, 7, 2, 4, 6

Rank the numbers in ascending order:

   2
   3
   4
   5
   6
   7

The median value is 4.5, the average of the third and fourth numbers.

Mode

The third indicator of central tendency is the *mode*. This is the number that occurs most frequently in a group of numbers.

PROBLEMS

What is the modal number for the following group of numbers?

   35, 34, 32, 40, 36, 33, 32, 31

The first step is to arrange the numbers from lowest to highest:

Lowest 31
      32
      32
      33
      34

                    35
                    36
        Highest 40

Next, determine which number or numbers occur most frequently:

Number	Frequency
31	1
32	2
33	1
34	1
35	1
36	1
40	1

From this chart, you can see that the number 32 occurs two times. Therefore, 32 is the modal number for this group of numbers.

What is the modal number for this group of numbers?

    104, 110, 120, 110, 115, 118, 107, 110, 108, 119, 106

To determine the modal number, arrange the numbers in order from lowest to highest:

    Lowest 104
            106
            107
            108
            110
            110
            110
            115
            118
            119
    Highest 120

Next, determine the frequency of each number:

Number	Frequency
104	1
106	1
107	1
108	1
110	3
115	1
118	1
119	1
120	1

From this chart, it can be determined that 110 is the modal number.

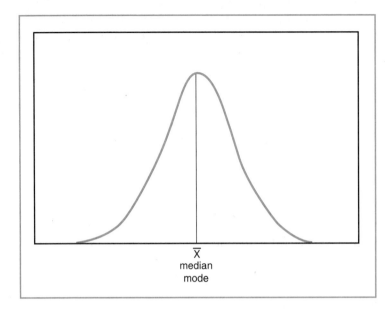

$\overline{X}$
median
mode

FIGURE 13-1 Gaussian distribution. (From Doucette, L. J. [1997]. *Mathematics for the Clinical Laboratory* [p. 259]. Philadelphia: W.B. Saunders Company.)

Gaussian Distribution

The mean, median, and mode are all indicators of central tendency. When these indicators are all the same number, we say that the group of numbers has a *Gaussian* distribution. Figure 13-1 shows a Gaussian distribution. A synonym for Gaussian distribution is *normal* distribution. A Gaussian distribution is bell-shaped, with an equal number of values above and below the highest point of the bell. Most statistics used in the laboratory assume that the data have a Gaussian distribution. This may or may not be true in all areas of health care. For example, statistics used in research may not have a Gaussian distribution. In this situation, non-Gaussian statistical methods must be used for data analysis. Population statistics may or may not have a Gaussian distribution as well. In a Gaussian distribution, since the mean, median, and mode are equal, a frequency distribution of the data would have a bell shape.

Accuracy versus Precision

Laboratory test results are often used initially to assess a patient's condition and determine a treatment plan; subsequently, they are used to monitor the patient's condition. Therefore, it is vital that these test results be of the highest quality. Two statistical terms are used to describe the quality of the result produced by the clinical laboratory: *accuracy* and *precision*. An accurate result is one that correctly reflects the true value of the result. Imagine a target value that should be obtained for an analyte.

If the results obtained have the target value, we can say that the results are accurate. The mean value of the data should be very close to the target value. In the laboratory, quality assurance methods are used to ensure that the results are centrally located, i.e., that they hit the target.

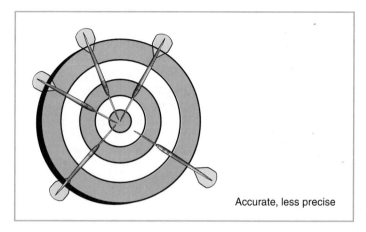

Accurate, less precise

Precision occurs when, after repeated analysis, the same result is achieved. Precision is related to the amount of dispersion of the data around the target value. If there is a great deal of dispersion, the results are not precise. Precise results are those that are tightly clustered together. Laboratory values should be tightly clustered around the true value, i.e., both accurate and precise. The statistical tools of variance, standard deviation, and coefficient of variation help assess the degree of dispersion of the data. The variance and standard deviation are commonly used to determine the acceptable range of quality control values that the laboratory will use, and the coefficient of variation is used to compare the precision of two different instruments. The more precise an instrument is, the more likely that the values obtained from that instrument will be accurate as well. In addition, the Clinical Laboratory Improvement Amendment of 1988 requires laboratories that perform moderate- and high-complexity tests to engage in proficiency testing (PT) to evaluate the quality of their results. Using an instrument that is very precise will decrease the chance of PT failure due to a result that falls outside of the acceptable range. More information on PT can be found in Chapter 15.

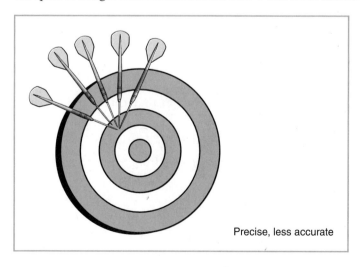

Precise, less accurate

Variance

The precision of a group of numbers is indicated by the *variance*. The symbol for variance is s^2. The variance indicates how far apart from each other, or how precise, are the numbers within a group. A group of numbers with a large variance would be expected to have a wide range of values. A group of numbers with a small variance would be expected to have a narrow range of values. The smaller the variance of a group of numbers, the more precise they are. Variance is calculated using the following formula:

$$s^2 = \frac{\Sigma(X_d - \overline{X})^2}{n - 1}$$

where

s^2 = variance
Σ = the sum of the numbers within parentheses
X_d = an individual data point within the group
$\overline{X}$ = the mean of the group of numbers
n = the total quantity of numbers within the group

Most scientific calculators have a variance function. By using the statistical mode of the calculator, the variance can be easily obtained. Manually caculating the variance of a group of numbers is time-consuming but may be necessary if a scientific calculator is not available.

To calculate the variance of a group of numbers, first determine the mean of the group. Then, subtract the mean from each number in the group. Sometimes a negative number will result if the mean is lower than a particular number in the group. Each product of the subtraction of the mean is then squared. The next step is to determine the sum of the individually squared numbers. This value is the numerator of the formula and is divided by the total quantity of numbers in the group $(n) - 1$. The number obtained from this calculation is the variance of the group. The units associated with the variance value will also be squared and will be different from the units of the group of numbers for which the variance was calculated.

PROBLEMS

Calculate the variance of the following group of total cholesterol values (in mg/dL):

185, 183, 182, 190, 191, 183, 185, 188, 189, 187

To calculate the variance, first rank the numbers from highest to lowest:

Lowest 182
       183
       183
       185
       185

187

188

189

190

Highest 191

Next, find the mean of the group of numbers by first determining the sum of the set of numbers:

182 + 183 + 183 + 185 + 185 + 187 + 188 + 189 + 190 + 191 = 1863 mg/dL

Therefore, the sum, or Σ, of this set of numbers is 1863 mg/dL.

Next, divide the sum by n:

$$\frac{1863}{10 \text{ or } n} = 186.3 \quad \text{or} \quad 186 \text{ mg/dL}$$

Now, subtract the mean, 186 mg/dL, from each of the numbers in the set:

Column 1 (Cholesterol, mg/dL)	Column 2 $(X_d - \overline{X})$
182	182 − 186 = −4
183	183 − 186 = −3
183	183 − 186 = −3
185	185 − 186 = −1
185	185 − 186 = −1
187	187 − 186 = +1
188	188 − 186 = +2
189	189 − 186 = +3
190	190 − 186 = +4
191	191 − 186 = +5

Next, square the difference obtained in column 2:

Column 1 (Cholesterol, mg/dL)	Column 2 $(X_d - \overline{X})$	Column 3 $(X_d - \overline{X})^2$
182	182 − 186 = −4	$(-4)^2 = 16$
183	183 − 186 = −3	$(-3)^2 = 9$
183	183 − 186 = −3	$(-3)^2 = 9$
185	185 − 186 = −1	$(-1)^2 = 1$
185	185 − 186 = −1	$(-1)^2 = 1$
187	187 − 186 = +1	$(+1)^2 = 1$
188	188 − 186 = +2	$(+2)^2 = 4$
189	189 − 186 = +3	$(+3)^2 = 9$
190	190 − 186 = +4	$(+4)^2 = 16$
191	191 − 186 = +5	$(+5)^2 = 25$

Now, find the sum of the numbers obtained in column 3:

16 + 9 + 9 + 1 + 1 + 1 + 4 + 9 + 16 + 25 = 91

Using the variance formula, substitute into it the numbers calculated so far:

$$s^2 = \frac{\Sigma(X_d - \overline{X})^2}{n - 1}$$

$$= \frac{91}{9} = 10 \text{ mg}^2/\text{dL}^2$$

The variance for this group of cholesterol values is 10 mg^2/dL^2.

Calculate the variance for the following group of total bilirubin values (in mg/dL):

1.2, 0.9, 0.8, 1.4, 1.5, 0.8

First, rank the numbers in order from lowest to highest:

0.8, 0.8, 0.9, 1.2, 1.4, 1.5

Next, determine the mean for the group of numbers:

0.8 + 0.8 + 0.9 + 1.2 + 1.4 + 1.5 = Σ = 6.6

The number 6.6 is divided by the n value of 6 to determine the mean of this group of numbers: 1.1 mg/dL. Now subtract the mean, 1.1 mg/dL, from each of the numbers in the set.

Column 1	Column 2
(Bilirubin, mg/dL)	$(X_d - \overline{X})$
0.8	0.8 − 1.1 = −0.3
0.8	0.8 − 1.1 = −0.3
0.9	0.9 − 1.1 = −0.2
1.2	1.2 − 1.1 = +0.1
1.4	1.4 − 1.1 = +0.3
1.5	1.5 − 1.1 = +0.4

Next, square the difference obtained in column 2:

Column 1	Column 2	Column 3
(Bilirubin, mg/dL)	$(X_d - \overline{X})$	$(X_d - \overline{X})^2$
0.8	0.8 − 1.1 = −0.3	0.09
0.8	0.8 − 1.1 = −0.3	0.09
0.9	0.9 − 1.1 = −0.2	0.04
1.2	1.2 − 1.1 = +0.1	0.01
1.4	1.4 − 1.1 = +0.3	0.09
1.5	1.5 − 1.1 = +0.4	0.16

Now, find the sum of the numbers obtained in column 3:

0.09 + 0.09 + 0.04 + 0.01 + 0.09 + 0.16 = 0.48

Using the variance formula, substitute into it the numbers calculated so far:

$$s^2 = \frac{\Sigma(X_d - \overline{X})^2}{n - 1}$$

$$= \frac{0.48}{5} = 0.096 \ \text{mg}^2/\text{dL}^2$$

The variance for this group of bilirubin values is 0.096 mg^2/dL^2.

Standard Deviation

In the clinical laboratory, the *standard deviation* is the most frequently used measure of precision. Its symbol is *s*. The standard deviation is the square root of the variance. Note that the units of measurement for the variance are also squared. By taking the square root of the variance, one expresses the units in the same terms as the mean, median, and mode.

PROBLEMS

Using the same group of cholesterol values (185, 183, 182, 190, 191, 183, 185, 188, 189, 187) used to calculate a variance, calculate the standard deviation.

The formula for the standard deviation is:

$$s = \sqrt{\frac{\Sigma(X_d - \overline{X}^2}{n - 1}}$$

The variance calculated in the previous example was 10 mg^2/dL^2.

$$s = \sqrt{10 \ \text{mg}^2/\text{dL}^2}$$
$$= 3.2 \ \text{mg/dL}$$

This group of cholesterol values has a standard deviation of 3.2 mg/dL. This means that within this group of numbers, the numbers deviate from the central value, or mean, by an average of 3.2 mg/dL. This deviation is referred to as *plus/minus (or ±) 1 standard deviation*. The smaller the standard deviation of a group of numbers, the closer together the numbers are in value and the higher the precision of the group of numbers. Conversely, the larger the standard deviation of a group of numbers, the further apart the numbers are and the lower the precision of the group of numbers.

Using the same group of bilirubin values (1.2, 0.9, 0.8, 1.4, 1.5, 0.8) used to calculate a variance, calculate the standard deviation.

The formula for the standard deviation is:

$$s = \sqrt{\frac{\Sigma(X_d - \overline{X})^2}{n - 1}}$$

The variance calculated in the previous example was 0.096 mg^2/dL^2. The standard deviation of 0.096 mg^2/dL^2 is:

$$s = \sqrt{0.096 \ \text{mg}^2/\text{dL}^2}$$
$$= 0.31 \ \text{mg/dL}$$

Therefore, the standard deviation for the group of bilirubin values is 0.31 mg/dL.

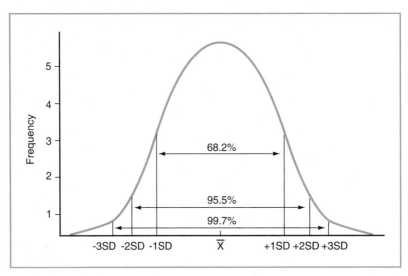

FIGURE 13-2 Probabilities associated with standard deviations. (From Doucette, L. J. [1997]. *Mathematics for the Clinical Laboratory* [p. 263]. Philadelphia: W.B. Saunders Company.)

Probabilities Associated with Standard Deviation

Statistically, if a sample is analyzed 30 times and the mean and standard deviation are established for the results obtained, then 68.2% of the time the results will fall within ±1 standard deviation from the mean, 95.5% of the time the results will fall within ±2 standard deviations from the mean, and 99.7% of the time the results will fall within ±3 standard deviations from the mean. This concept is shown in Figure 13-2. These statistical probabilities are used when establishing the acceptable limits of quality control results.

PROBLEMS

If the mean for glucose in a quality control material is 80 mg/dL and 1 standard deviation is 5 mg/dL, what is the probability that if the control material is reanalyzed, the result will fall between 75 and 85 mg/dL (±1 standard deviation)?

Statistically, it is known that 68.2% of the time a result will fall within ±1 standard deviation of an established value (mean). In this case, if the sample was analyzed 100 times, then in 68 analyses the results will be between 75 and 85 mg/dL. On the other hand, 32 of the analyses will fall outside of this range.

If the mean for the total white blood cell count in a quality control material is determined to be 9000 mm³ and the standard deviation for the method is determined to be 100 mm³, what is the statistical chance that a sample of this quality control material will fall within the laboratory's quality control guideline of ±2 standard deviations, or, in other words, between 8900 and 9100 mm³?

Statistically, there is a 95% chance that if this control material is tested, the result will fall within a range of 8900 to 9100 mm³.

Establishing Standard Deviation Ranges, Standard Deviation Intervals, or Confidence Intervals

Before using a new lot number (or batch) of quality control material for each test that is performed in a laboratory, it is good practice for each laboratory to determine its own standard deviation range for every test performed, using all levels of quality control materials, instead of relying on the values provided by the manufacturer. This is because there may be differences in instrument performance or laboratory environment that may impact the laboratory values. By establishing its own values, the laboratory will be able to assess more accurately where the majority of quality control results will fall and will be able to determine more accurately when quality control results are truly out of control.

The terms *standard deviation range, standard deviation interval,* and *confidence limits* have the same meaning. For clarity, the term *standard deviation range* will be used to explain the concept. The standard deviation range is a measurement of *dispersion*. It is calculated by subtracting the standard deviation value from the mean value to establish the lowest number in the range and by adding the standard deviation value to the mean value to establish the highest number in the range. Thus, the standard deviation range is the range of numbers from lowest to highest that are clustered or dispersed around the mean. Standard deviation ranges are established for quality control material by each laboratory as a method of setting acceptable quality control limits. Frequently, 1, 2, and 3 standard deviation ranges are established.

PROBLEMS

Twenty replicates of a single bottle of quality control material were analyzed for hemoglobin. The mean hemoglobin value was found to be 15.0 mg/dL. The standard deviation was calculated to be 2.2 mg/dL. What would be the 1, 2, and 3 standard deviation ranges, or confidence intervals, for the quality control?

To establish the standard deviation range, the standard deviation value is both subtracted from and added to the mean value to establish the lower and upper limits of the range, respectively. The 1 standard deviation range is established as follows:

$$1 \text{ standard deviation} = 2.2 \text{ mg/dL; mean} = 15.0 \text{ mg/dL}$$
$$15.0 - 2.2 = 12.8 \text{ mg/dL}$$
$$15.0 + 2.2 = 17.2 \text{ mg/dL}$$

The 1 standard deviation range is 12.8–17.2 mg/dL. This means that all numbers falling between 12.8 and 17.2 mg/dL are within 1 standard deviation of the mean.

$$2 \text{ standard deviations} = 1 \text{ standard deviation} \times 2 = 2.2 \times 2 = 4.4 \text{ mg/dL}$$
$$15.0 - 4.4 = 10.6 \text{ mg/dL}$$
$$15.0 + 4.4 = 19.4 \text{ mg/dL}$$

The 2 standard deviation range is 10.6–19.4 mg/dL. Therefore, all numbers falling between 10.6 and 19.4 mg/dL are within 2 standard deviations of the mean.

$$3 \text{ standard deviations} = 1 \text{ standard deviation} \times 3 = 2.2 \times 3 = 6.6 \text{ mg/dL}$$
$$15.0 - 6.6 = 8.4 \text{ mg/dL}$$
$$15.0 + 6.6 = 21.6 \text{ mg/dL}$$

The 3 standard deviation range is 8.4–21.6 mg/dL. Therefore, all numbers falling between 8.4 and 21.6 mg/dL are within 3 standard deviations of the mean.

If the mean for a group of cholesterol quality control values is 220 mg/dL and the standard deviation for the method is 4 mg/dL, what are the ±1, 2, and 3 standard deviation ranges for this control?

The +1 standard deviation value is determined by adding 4 to 220, or 224. The −1 standard deviation value is determined by subtracting 4 from 220, or 216. Therefore, the ±1 standard deviation range is from 216 to 224 mg/dL.

The +2 and −2 standard deviation range is calculated as follows:

$$220 + 8 = 228$$
$$220 - 8 = 212$$

Therefore, the ±2 standard deviation range is from 212 to 228 mg/dL.

The ±3 standard deviation range is calculated as follows:

$$220 + 12 = 232$$
$$220 - 12 = 208$$

Therefore, the ±3 standard deviation range is from 208 to 232 mg/dL.

Coefficient of Variation

The last statistical term used to describe dispersion or precision is the *coefficient of variation* (*CV*). It is useful when comparing two or more groups of data to determine which has the greatest precision. The lower the CV for a group of data, the more precise the data. The CV is calculated by the following formula:

$$\%CV = \frac{s}{\overline{X}} \times 100$$

The CV is expressed as a percentage.

PROBLEMS

If a glucose method had a mean control value of 85 mg/dL and a standard deviation of 2 mg/dL, what is the CV for this method?

Using the CV formula, the following calculation is derived:

$$\%CV = \frac{2.0 \text{ mg/dL}}{85 \text{ mg/dL}} \times 100 = 2.4\%$$

The CV for this glucose method is 2.4%.

A medical laboratory technician is evaluating a new cholesterol instrument for the physician's office laboratory where she works. The current cholesterol instrument has a CV of 2.4%, and the CV for the new instrument is 1.8%. Which method is more precise?

Since the lower the CV of a group of numbers the higher the precision of the numbers, the new cholesterol instrument should be more precise than the current instrument.

EXAMPLE PROBLEMS

This section is designed to be useful to both the student and the health care practitioner. Students can use the example problems in order to master the material. The health care practitioner can use these problems as templates for performing laboratory calculations. Find an example problem similar to the problem that you need to solve and substitute into the equation the numbers appropriate to your calculation.

1. **Q What is the mean of the following set of numbers?**
   14, 18, 16, 13, 11, 19, 20, 10, 18, 13

   A The mean of a group of numbers is calculated by adding the numbers and dividing the sum by the total quantity of numbers in the set. In this problem there are 10 numbers, and their sum is 152. The mean is calculated by dividing this number by 10, resulting in a mean of 15.2, which is rounded to 15.

2. **Q What is the mean of the following set of numbers?**
   25.7, 26.8, 32.2, 40.4, 29.1, 26.8

   A The mean of this set of numbers is 31.8.

3. **Q What is the median of the following set of numbers?**
   2.62, 2.62, 2.56, 2.58, 2.60, 2.61, 2.64

A The median number is the number in the middle of a group of ranked numbers. An even number of digits is above and below the median number in a set of numbers. To calculate the median number, first rank the numbers in order from lowest to highest:

2.56, 2.58, 2.60, 2.61, 2.62, 2.62, 2.64.

Since the total quantity of numbers in the set is an odd number, seven, add 1 to the total quantity of numbers and divide the sum by 2. In this case, 7 + 1 = 8, and 8 ÷ 2 = 4. Finally, find the fourth number in the list of numbers. In this case it is 2.61.

2.56, 2.58, 2.60, 2.61, 2.62, 2.62, 2.64.

Note that the median number is the middle number in the group and that there is an equal number of digits above and below the median number.

4. **Q** **What is the median number of this set of numbers?**

85, 77, 87, 78, 79, 80, 82

A The median number of this set of numbers is 80:

77, 78, 79, 80, 82, 85, 87.

5. **Q** **What is the median number of this set of numbers?**

258, 237, 241, 250, 260, 248, 238, 245, 256, 246

A The first step is to rank the numbers in order from lowest to highest:

237, 238, 241, 245, 246, 248, 250, 256, 256, 260

This set is composed of 10 numbers, an even number. In this case, to find the median, first divide the total quantity of the set of numbers, in this case 10, by 2, resulting in the number 5. Next, add 1 to the number 5: 5 + 1 = 6. The median value for this set of numbers is the *average* of the fifth and sixth numbers.

237
238
241
245
246 fifth number
248 sixth number
250
256
256
260

The average of 246 and 248 is 247. Therefore, the median number for this set of numbers is 247. Note that there is an equal quantity of digits above and below the median value.

6. **Q** **What is the median value for this set of numbers?**
135, 128, 132, 134, 129, 131

A The median value for this set of numbers is 131.5, the average of the third and fourth numbers.
128, 129, 131, *131.5*, 132, 134, 135

7. **Q** **Determine the modal number for this set of numbers:**
498, 480, 484, 479, 488, 487, 482, 487, 487, 490, 492, 491

A The modal number, or mode, is the number in a set of numbers that occurs most frequently. In a Gaussian distribution, there is only one modal number. In other distribution patterns there may be more than one modal number. The modal number is calculated by first ranking the numbers from lowest to highest:
479, 480, 482, 484, 487, 487, 487, 488, 490, 491, 492, 498
Next, determine the frequency of occurrence for each number:

Number	Frequency
479	1
480	1
482	1
484	1
487	3
488	1
490	1
491	1
492	1
498	1

The modal number is the number that occurs most frequently. The frequency chart shows that 487 occurs three times, while all other numbers occur only once. Therefore, the modal number for this group of numbers is 487.

8. **Q** **What is the modal number for this set of numbers?**
53, 56, 57, 53, 52, 58, 57, 53, 56, 53

A The modal number for this set of numbers is 53, which occurs four times. Other numbers within this set occur more than once, but none occurs as many as four times.

9. **Q** **Calculate the variance of this set of numbers:**
295, 290, 298, 287, 291, 301, 303, 300

A The variance can be calculated by two methods. The first, and faster method, is with a scientific calculator using the statistical mode. Because scientific calculators vary in keystrokes, consult the manufacturer's instructions on how to use this function. The second method involves manual calculation. First, determine the total quantity of numbers, or n. In this example there are eight numbers, so $n = 8$. Next, determine the mean of the set of numbers. In this case, the mean value is 296. Next, rank the numbers from lowest to highest and subtract the mean, 296, from each number. The term X_d denotes each digit in this set of numbers.

Column 1	Column 2
287	$287 - 296 = -9$
290	$290 - 296 = -6$
291	$291 - 296 = -5$
295	$295 - 296 = -1$
298	$298 - 296 = +2$
300	$300 - 296 = +4$
301	$301 - 296 = +5$
303	$303 - 296 = +7$

Next, square the difference in column 2 and determine the sum of the numbers in column 3:

Column 1 (X_d)	Column 2 $(X_d - \overline{X})$	Column 3 $(X_d - \overline{X})^2$
287	-9	81
290	-6	36
291	-5	25
295	-1	1
298	$+2$	4
300	$+4$	16
301	$+5$	25
303	$+7$	49
		$\Sigma = 237$

Using the variance formula, substitute into it the numbers calculated so far:

$$s^2 = \frac{\Sigma(X_d - \overline{X})^2}{n - 1} = \frac{237}{7}$$

$$= 33.8.$$

Therefore, the variance for this set of numbers is 33.8.

10. Q Using the data from example problem 9, calculate the standard deviation of the set of numbers.

   A The standard deviation is the square root of the variance. Since the variance is 33.8, the square root of 33.8 is 5.8. Therefore, the standard deviation, or average precision, of this group of numbers is 5.8.

11. Q **Calculate the variance for the following group of hematocrit values in mg/dL:**

35.5, 40.0, 37.5, 36.0, 35.0, 38.0, 39.5, 34.5

A The mean for this group of numbers is 37.0 mg/dL. The n value is 8, as there are eight numbers in the group. The variance for this group of numbers is 2.1 mg^2/dL^2. Note that the units are squared for the variance value.

12. Q **Given the variance value from example problem 11, what is the standard deviation of this group of hematocrit values?**

A The standard deviation is the square root of the variance. The square root of 2.1 is 1.4. The units will now be expressed in their original form. Therefore, the standard deviation of this group of hematocrit values is 1.4 mg/dL.

13. Q **What is the probability that a quality control result will fall within ±1 standard deviation from the mean?**

A The probability that a quality control result will fall within ±1 standard deviation from the mean is 68.2%.

14. Q **What is the probability that a quality control result will fall outside of ±2 standard deviations from the mean?**

A The probability that a quality control result will fall outside of ±2 standard deviations from the mean is 4.5% or approximately 5%. This is because the probability that a quality control result will fall within ±2 standard deviations is 95.5%, meaning that if a quality control sample is measured 100 times, approximately 95 results will fall within the ±2 standard deviation range, while 5% will fall outside of the range.

15. Q **What is the probability that a quality control result will fall within the ±3 standard deviation range?**

A The probability that a result will fall within the ±3 standard deviation range is 99.7%. Therefore, there is only a 0.3% chance that a result that falls outside of this range is valid.

16. Q **Calculate the ±2 standard deviation range for the hematocrit results in example problem 11.**

A The mean of the group of numbers was calculated to be 37.0 mg/dL.

One standard deviation (SD) was calculated to be 1.4 mg/dL. Therefore, 2 standard deviations would be twice the value of 1 standard deviation, or 2.8 mg/dL (1.4 × 2). The ±2 standard deviation range from the mean is calculated by both adding to and subtracting the 2 standard deviation value from the mean. Therefore:

±2 SD = 37.0 + 1.4 = 38.4 mg/dL
−2 SD = 37.0 − 1.4 = 35.6 mg/dL

Therefore, the ±2 standard deviation range for this group of hematocrit values is from 35.6 mg/dL to 38.4 mg/dL.

17. **Q** **A new lot of high-level quality control material was assayed 30 times for cholesterol to establish the acceptable quality control limits. The mean of the cholesterol values was 265 mg/dL. The standard deviation was 5.5 mg/dL. Calculate the ±3 standard deviation range for cholesterol on this lot of control material.**

A The ±3 standard deviation range is calculated by first determining the value of 3 standard deviations. One standard deviation is equal to 5.5 mg/dL. Therefore, 3 standard deviations would be 3 times 5.5 mg/dL, or 16.5 mg/dL. Therefore, the 3 standard deviation range would be calculated by adding 16.5 mg/dL to the mean, 265 mg/dL, to determine the highest value in the range and subtracting 16.5 mg/dL from the mean of 265 mg/dL to determine the lowest value in the range:

±3 SD = 265 + 16.5 = 281.5 mg/dL
−3 SD = 265 − 16.5 = 248.5 mg/dL

Therefore, the ±3 standard deviation range for cholesterol analysis for this level of quality control material includes all values between 248.5 and 281.5 mg/dL.

18. **Q** **Calculate the CV for a group of quality control results assayed for glucose. The mean value is 450 mg/dL, and the standard deviation is 15 mg/dL.**

A The CV is calculated by the following formula:

$$CV = \frac{s}{\overline{X}} \times 100$$

The CV is expressed as a percentage. By substituting into the equation the values from the problem, the following equation is derived:

$$CV = \frac{15 \text{ mg/dL}}{450 \text{ mg/dL}} \times 100$$
$$= 3.3\%.$$

Therefore, the CV for this set of glucose results is 3.3%.

19. **Q** A new supervisor performs 30 replicate white blood cell determinations on the same tube of blood on two different hematology analyzers. The CV of the determinations on analyzer A is 1.4%, and the CV of the determinations on analyzer B is 2.0%. Which analyzer is more precise?

A The CV is a measurement of the precision of a method. The smaller the CV, the more precise the method. CV measurements do not reveal anything about the accuracy of the method. When two methods are compared, the method with the smaller CV is more precise. Therefore, in this comparison, analyzer A, which has a smaller CV than analyzer B, yields results that are more precise.

PRACTICE PROBLEMS

Solve the following practice problems to further master the material. All answers and explanations to some problems can be found in a separate section at the back of the book.

Given this set of numbers, solve the following problems:
45, 49, 43, 49, 51, 50, 47, 48
1. Calculate the mean for the set.
2. Calculate the median number in the set.
3. Calculate the modal number in the set.
4. Calculate the variance for the set.
5. Calculate the standard deviation of the set.
6. Calculate the CV of the set.

Given the following set of glucose results, solve the following problems:
420 mg/dL, 430 mg/dL, 425 mg/dL, 430 mg/dL, 429 mg/dL, 427 mg/dL, 433 mg/dL
7. Calculate the mean for the set.
8. Calculate the median glucose value.
9. Calculate the modal glucose value.
10. Calculate the variance for the set.
11. Calculate the standard deviation for the set.
12. Calculate the CV of the set.

List the probabilities associated with each event:
13. A control result falls within ±1 standard deviation of the mean.
14. A control result falls within ±2 standard deviations of the mean.

15. A control result falls within ±3 standard deviations of the mean.
16. A control result falls outside of ±2 standard deviations of the mean.
17. A control result falls outside of ±3 standard deviations of the mean.
18. If a group of data has a standard deviation of 1.5 and a mean value of 12.5, calculate the ±2 standard deviation range for the data.
19. If a group of data has a standard deviation of 10.5 and a mean value of 225, calculate the ±3 standard deviation range for the data.

BIBLIOGRAPHY

Burtis, C. A., and Ashwood, E. R. *Tietz Textbook of Clinical Chemistry,* 3rd ed. W.B. Saunders Company, Philadelphia, 1999.

Doucette, L. J. *Mathematics for the Clinical Laboratory.* W.B. Saunders Company, Philadelphia, 1997.

Glantz, A. *Primer of Biostatistics.* McGraw-Hill, Inc., New York, 1992.

Shot, S. *Statistics for Health Professionals.* W.B. Saunders Company, Philadelphia, 1990.

CHAPTER 14

Quality Assurance and Quality Control in the Clinical Laboratory

OBJECTIVES

Upon completion of this chapter, the reader should be able to:

1 Define the following terms: quality assurance, quality control material, preanalytical, analytical, and postanalytical errors, outlier, shift, trend, bias.

2 Plot quality control results on a Levey-Jennings chart.

3 Compare and contrast systematic and random errors.

4 Identify systematic and random errors.

5 Evaluate quality control results using Westgard multirules.

INTRODUCTION

Quality Assurance Concepts

In the laboratory, instruments and methodologies must be monitored to ensure accurate results. *Quality Assurance* is the process by which this occurs.

It consists of monitoring any activity associated with a laboratory result. Activities that occur before the sample reaches the laboratory are called *preanalytical* activities, those that occur in the laboratory and deal directly with analysis of the sample are called *analytical activities*, and those that occur after the analysis is performed are called *postanalytical activities*. Each of these types of activities must be monitored for errors to ensure accurate results. For example, if the wrong patient is drawn, that is a preanalytical error. If the sample is analyzed incorrectly, that is an analytical error. If the results are written on the wrong patient's chart, that is a postanalytical error. One technique that can be used to check quality assurance procedures is to follow random samples as they proceed from collection to analysis to charting of the results. By evaluating the progress of the samples throughout the entire testing process, errors in the quality assurance process can be determined and corrective action taken. Under the Clinical Laboratory Improvement Amendment of 1988 (CLIA'88), quality assurance activities in laboratories that perform moderate- or high-complexity testing must be evaluated on a continuing basis to ensure accurate results. It is considered good practice for laboratories that perform waived testing to also establish quality assurance procedures and protocols.

Quality Control Material

Within the laboratory, one method used to ensure the analytical quality of the patient results is to use quality control material. Quality control material is analyzed along with patient specimens and should be treated the same way as patient specimens. Quality control material should have the same chemical and physical properties as the patient sample. For example, if analytes in serum are measured, a serum-based quality control material should be used; if analytes in urine specimens are measured, a urine-based quality control material should be used. Quality control material is usually manufactured to contain many different analytes so that it can be used on multitest analyzers. The concentration of the analytes varies, depending on how many levels of quality control material the manufacturer puts in the assay. When two or more levels of quality control material are included in an assay, one level has the concentration of the analyte found in the normal population. The second level has either the elevated or a decreased concentration of the analyte and represents an abnormal control. Whether the second control has an elevated or decreased concentration of the analyte depends on the medical usefulness of the particular concentration. Some forms of testing require three levels of control to be analyzed because both the decreased and elevated levels of the analyte are medically useful. For example, when analyzing therapeutic drugs such as theophylline, three levels of control (low, medium, and high or 1, 2, and 3) are used. Under the rules of CLIA'88, at least two levels of quality control material must be included for every assay at least once a day (24 hours) or once per shift (every 8 hours) if there is more than one shift.[1]

Prior to patient testing and result reporting, as mandated by CLIA'88, the mean and standard deviation for each analyte are established for each level of quality control material. In this manner, the entire method can be monitored for errors, since whatever happens to the patient samples also happens to the quality control samples. For example, if the wrong pipette is used in an analysis and twice as much serum is used as was called for in the procedure, the results for the quality control samples will be twice as high as they should be. Without quality control material to check the accuracy of the method, errors can occur. If the quality control results fall outside of the laboratory's established range of acceptable results, the patient sample results cannot be reported until the cause of the unacceptable result is determined and corrected, and the quality control results are within acceptable limits.

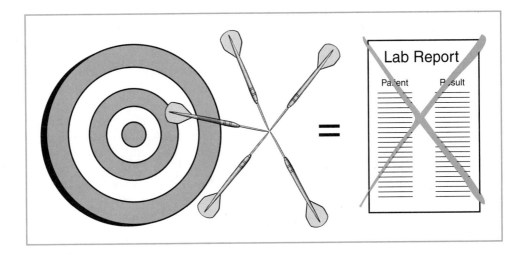

Quality control material may be in one of three forms. Lyophilized, or freeze-dried, quality control material must be reconstituted with diluent before use. It is critical to use the correct diluent and the correct quantity of diluent to ensure accurate quality control material results. Common diluents for lyophilized controls include deionized or distilled water or a buffered solution. The quantity of diluent must be measured by a calibrated pipette, not a syringe. The most accurate pipette is a volummetric pipette. Be sure to always use a pipette bulb or another pipetting device while pipetting. *Never* pipette by mouth. Although syringes are often used to reconstitute powdered medications, they are not calibrated with sufficient precision to be used to reconstitute controls.

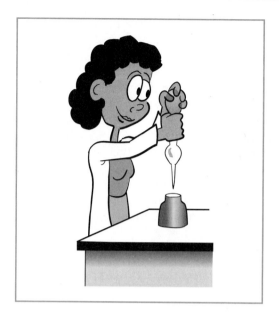

Lyophilized controls must also be allowed time to be fully reconstituted before use. Often this means that after the diluent is added, the control material is swirled gently to mix the diluent and lyophilized material, then left undisturbed for approximately 5–20 minutes to allow all of the lyophilized material to go into solution. If this timed process is not followed and the quality control material is used immediately after the diluent is added, inaccurate results may occur.

The second form of quality control material comes from the manufacturer prediluted and ready for use. No reconstitution is necessary for this type of control. The third type of material is ethylene-glycol-based controls. These controls are prediluted in ethylene glycol and should not be used on analytes measured by ion specific electrodes, as the ethylene glycol may damage the electrodes. Ethylene-glycol controls are stored in liquid form at 0°C.

Quality Control Analysis

After quality control materials are used, the results of the analysis must be evaluated before patient results are reported to the physician. There are many different evaluation methods for quality control results; a complete list is beyond the scope of this book. The basic statistical concepts discussed in Chapter 13 form the basis for quality control analysis. Recall that 68.2% of the time a control result will fall within ±1 standard deviation of the mean, 95.5% of the time the results will fall within ±2 standard deviations of the mean, and 99.7% of the time the results will fall within ±3 standard deviations of the mean. On the other hand, approximately 32% of the time the results will fall outside of the ±1 standard deviation interval, almost 5% of the time they will fall outside of the ±2 standard deviation interval, and 0.3% of the time they will fall outside of the ±3 standard deviation interval. These statistical probabilities are used when establishing the acceptable limits of quality control results.

The question that the health care practitioner has to ask and answer is: What are the acceptable limits for the quality control material used? Remember, if the quality control result is outside of the acceptable limits established by the laboratory, the patient results cannot be reported until the problem is solved. If a laboratory uses the 2 standard deviation range as its acceptable limit, then 5 times out of 100 or 1 time out of 20, the results will fall outside of accepted limits by chance alone. This means that if a result falls outside 2 standard deviations, there is a 95% chance that it is invalid and only a 5% chance that it is valid and fell outside of the range simply by chance. Quality control results that fall outside of the acceptable range are called *outliers*. The test system is termed *out of control*, and action must be taken to determine the cause of the outliers. Good laboratory practice dictates that all corrective actions are documented and patient results not reported until the method is in control.

Figure 14-1*A* is a chart of quality control results for level I glucose control for the month of May obtained by a small clinic. Figure 14-1*B* is the corrective action log for the laboratory. Note the notations on the corrective action log and how the individual control results are plotted on the chart.

Whether or not outlier control values should be included in the laboratory's quality control statistics depends on the laboratory's quality assurance protocol. In general, if the outlier value can be traced back to a problem with the control itself—for example, an outdated control—the outlier value is not included in the statistics.

In the hematology laboratory, the quality control technique of *moving averages* is used on automated analyzers to establish the control limits for the erythrocyte indices.[2] Erythrocyte indices within a given population tend to be stable. In the moving averages technique, 20 consecutive patient samples are batched and the mean is calculated by the instrument. An overall mean is established for every 20 batches of patient samples (400 different patients). This technique uses a complex mathematical formula to "smooth" the individual results within the batches, thereby allowing means and standard deviations to be calculated for each index. However, due to the large patient population required, this method of quality control is generally not used in small laboratories or in most physician office laboratories.

Errors That Cause a Method to Be out of Control

There are two main reasons why a method is out of control. The first is *random error* that occurs by chance. In the 2 standard deviation range, random error is

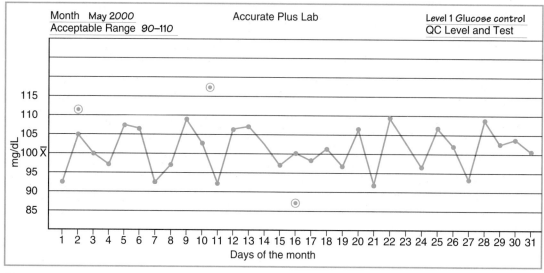

A

Accurate Plus Lab
Corrective Action Log

Date	Quality Assurance Problem
5/2/00	Level 1 Glucose out of range, (high)

Corrective Action Taken:
Repeat control.
Problem Corrected? (Yes) No
Additional Action and Follow-up
None

Date	Quality Assurance Problem
5/10/00	Level 1 Glucose out of range, (high)

Corrective Action Taken:
Repeat control.
Problem Corrected? (Yes) No
Additional Action and Follow-up
None

Date	Quality Assurance Problem
5/16/00	Level 1 Glucose out of range, (low)

Corrective Action Taken:
Make up new bottle of control, control near out-date.
Problem Corrected? (Yes) No
Additional Action and Follow-up
None

B

FIGURE 14-1 *A,* Level I glucose control for May 2000; *B,* Corrective Action Log.

why the results will be outside of the range 5 out of 100 times even though there is nothing wrong with the method. Health care professionals strive to keep random error as low as possible. An example of random error is a 100 μL pipette that delivers 100 μL of sample in most samples to be analyzed but delivers only 90 μL of sample in a few samples. Those few samples will have inaccurate results because insufficient sample was pipetted. Routine maintenance and calibration can reduce the chance of this random error. Random error is related to the precision of the test method.

The second type of error is *systematic error*. This type of error occurs, as the name implies, systematically; all samples are affected, not just a few. Systematic error may produce a *bias* in the method, causing the results to be artificially elevated or decreased. One cause of systematic error is a refrigerator that does not keep the reagents at the proper temperature. Reagents that contain enzymes will be affected, as the enzymes may lose their strength or activity if not stored properly. The results obtained for all of the samples and quality control material may be falsely lowered and inaccurate. Another systematic error is a method that is not properly calibrated. All results will be adversely affected in either a positive or negative direction. Systematic error can also occur if, instead of following the laboratory's procedure and using a 100 μL micropipette to deliver a sample, a 1 cc syringe is used to measure 0.1 cc of sample. It may be tempting to use syringes instead of pipettes when performing laboratory tests, but syringes are not calibrated as accurately as pipettes. Any initial time savings from using a syringe will probably be lost due to error if either over- or undersampling occurs. The chance of systematic error can be reduced by following written laboratory procedures, as well as proper calibration and routine maintenance of all laboratory equipment and instruments. Systematic error is related to the accuracy of the test method.

Levey-Jennings Charts

CLIA'88 and good laboratory practice require the use of at least two quality control materials for each method to ensure accurate and reliable patient results. The results of the quality control material analysis must be evaluated to determine if the method is in control before patient results are reported. One mechanism for quickly evaluating each control value is to plot the value on an individual Levey-Jennings Control Chart. This chart, as shown in Figure 14-2, consists of a graph in which the mean and standard deviation ranges are plotted on the y axis and the days of the month are plotted on the x axis. Each level of quality control material for a particular analyte has its own Levey-Jennings chart. For example, although CLIA'88 requires the use of only two levels of quality control material for automated hematology analyzers, many laboratories use three levels. For example, if the analyte was hemoglobin, the results obtained from the three different levels of controls would be plotted on three different Levey-Jennings charts, one chart for each level of control.

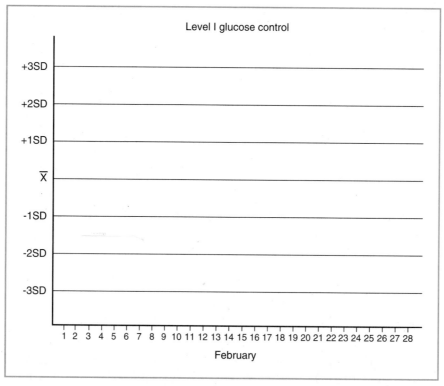

FIGURE 14-2 Levey-Jennings chart for level I glucose control. (From Doucette, L. J. [1997]. *Mathematics for the Clinical Laboratory* [p. 281]. Philadelphia: W.B. Saunders Company.)

PROBLEM

Three levels of control are run daily on an automated hematology analyzer in a physician's office laboratory. The mean for the normal level is 14 mg/dL, with a standard deviation of 1.2 mg/dL. What will the Levey-Jennings chart look like if a medical laboratory technician plotted, over a 5 day period, hemoglobin results obtained from the normal level of quality control material?

The hemoglobin results obtained are:

    day 1 = 13 mg/dL, day 2 = 12.5 mg/dL, day 3 = 16 mg/dL,
    day 4 = 15.3 mg/dL, day 5 = 14 mg/dL.

The Levey-Jennings chart consists of the days of the week or times of the run on the x axis and the mean and standard deviation intervals for the particular level of quality control material on the y axis. A *run* consists of the quality control material and patient samples analyzed during a time period when the test method is stable and no changes are made to the test method or instrumentation. Under CLIA'88, the maximum time frame for a run is 24 hours.

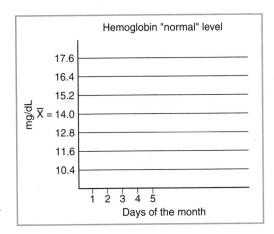

FIGURE 14-3 Levey-Jennings chart demonstrating hemoglobin normal levels.

To construct the Levey-Jennings chart, the 1, 2, and 3 standard deviation intervals must be calculated first. The mean for the level to be plotted is 14 mg/dL, and the standard deviation is 1.2 mg/dL. Therefore, the ±1 standard deviation interval will be 12.8 to 15.2 mg/dL, the ±2 standard deviation interval will be 11.6 to 16.4 mg/dL, and the ±3 standard deviation interval will be 10.4 to 17.6 mg/dL. These interval values are plotted on the y axis of the chart. The days of the run are plotted on the x axis. Figure 14-3 illustrates the Levey-Jennings chart up to this point.

Next, the five values obtained are plotted on the chart by placing a dot or circle at the intersection where the value is found on the y axis and the day analyzed on the x axis, as shown in Figure 14-4.

Last, each result obtained from the same lot number is connected to the next result by a line, as illustrated in Figure 14-5. When a new lot number is used, the mean and standard deviation may be different and should be recalculated before use in

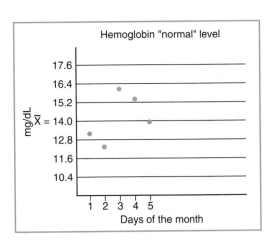

FIGURE 14-4 Levey-Jennings chart demonstrating hemoglobin normal levels.

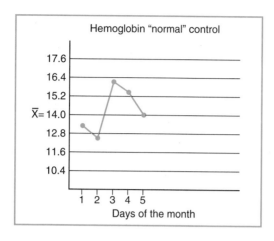

FIGURE 14-5 Levey-Jennings chart demonstrating hemoglobin normal controls.

patient sampling. Then, either a new Levey-Jennings chart is used, or the same Levey-Jennings chart is used but the results from the two different lot numbers are not connected by a line. A notation should be placed where the results from the new lot number begin to be charted.

Shifts and Trends

By plotting quality control results on a Levey-Jennings chart, shifts and trends in the quality control results can be quickly discovered. A *shift* is a sudden change (either an increase or a decrease) in the quality control results that causes the results to be distributed solely on one side or the other of the mean for 6 or 7 consecutive days. Shifts occur due to systematic error. A new lot of reagent may have inadvertently been used, or a method that is not calibrated can cause a shift to occur. Figure 14-6 demonstrates a shift on a Levey-Jennings chart of the low level of hemoglobin quality control material. When a shift occurs, the cause must be found and corrected because the method is out of control.

PROBLEM

The following quality control results obtained on days 6 through 11 for a normal level of control material for total cholesterol must be plotted on the Levey-Jennings chart (Figure 14-7). The results for days 1 through 5 have already been plotted.

day 6 = 180 mg/dL, day 7 = 185 mg/dL, day 8 = 182 mg/dL, day 9 = 181 mg/dL, day 10 = 181 mg/dL, day 11 = 182 mg/dL.

Is there anything wrong with these quality control results? If so, what are some of the predominant causes?

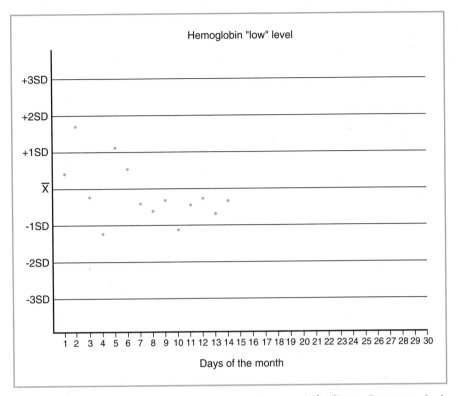

FIGURE 14-6 Levey-Jennings chart demonstrating a shift. (From Doucette, L. J. [1997]. *Mathematics for the Clinical Laboratory* [p. 284]. Philadelphia: W.B. Saunders Company.)

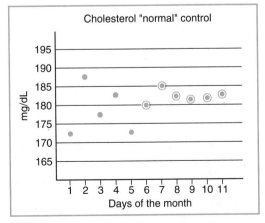

FIGURE 14-7 Levey-Jennings chart for normal level cholesterol control.

The quality control results demonstrate a shift. All the results fall on the same side of the mean, which is statistically unlikely, and there is an abrupt change in the pattern of the results. The most likely cause of the shift is a change in instrument temperature, another malfunction, or another type of systematic error.

A *trend* occurs when the quality control results gradually either decrease or increase over a period of 6 or 7 days. A trend is also due to systematic error, but the type of error tends to occur more slowly over time. For example, reagents stored in a refrigerator that is slowly becoming unable to keep the correct temperature may deteriorate over time. Figure 14-8 demonstrates a trend occurring in level II of a quality control material for automated white blood cell counts. As with shifts, when trends occur, the cause must be found and corrected.

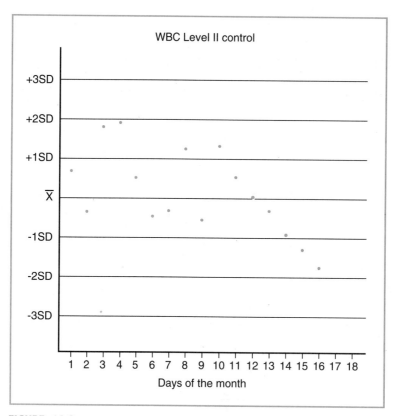

FIGURE 14-8 Levey-Jennings chart demonstrating a trend. (From Doucette, L. J. [1997]. *Mathematics for the Clinical Laboratory* [p. 287]. Philadelphia: W.B. Saunders Company.)

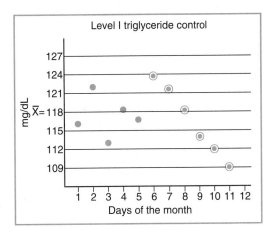

FIGURE 14-9 Levey-Jennings chart for level I triglyceride controls.

PROBLEM

Plot the following level I triglyceride quality control results for days 6 through 11 on the Levey-Jennings chart (Figure 14-9). Is there anything wrong with these results? If so, what could be the cause?

day 6 = 124 mg/dL, day 7 = 122 mg/dL, day 8 = 118 mg/dL,
day 9 = 114 mg/dL, day 10 = 112 mg/dL, day 11 = 109 mg/dL

These quality control results demonstrate a trend. Over the course of at least six runs, the results of the control show a consistent downturn in value. Statistically, this is not likely to occur. It is probably caused by a systematic error that is decreasing the triglyceride results slowly over time. One cause could be a malfunctioning refrigerator that is slowly losing its ability to cool sufficiently, thereby causing the triglyceride reagent to deteriorate and lose its activity.

Westgard Multirules

Each laboratory is responsible for establishing its own criteria for acceptance or rejection of quality control results. For some laboratories, this may mean using the ±2 standard deviation range as the cutoff point for accepting results. Any quality control results above or below 2 standard deviations are rejected, and the method is considered to be out of control. For most laboratories, this criterion is too stringent. Remember that approximately 5% of the time a valid result will fall outside of the 2 standard deviation range. Other laboratories may use a 2.5 standard deviation range as the cutoff. Today it is possible to program many laboratory instruments with the laboratory's control criterion. When a control result is outside of the criterion, it is *flagged* by the computer. Quality control

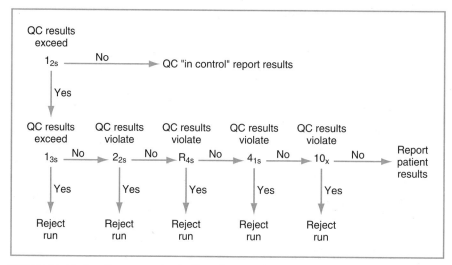

FIGURE 14-10 Quality control rule flow for two levels of controls. (Redrawn from Westgard, J. O., Barry, P. L., Hunt, M. R., and Groth, T. [1981]. A multi-rule Shewhart chart for quality control in clinical chemistry. *Clinical Chemistry*, 27:493–501.)

assessments including Levey-Jennings charts can be recalled by the computer on a daily or monthly basis.

In 1981, Westgard, Barry, and Hunt developed a set of quality control rules to interpret quality control results in the clinical laboratory.[3] Since CLIA'88 requires a minimum of two levels of control to be used for each method, the rules pertaining to two levels of control will be discussed next. Westgard has also developed a set of rules for interpreting control results.[4] These rules will not be discussed, as the complexity of the use and interpretation of these rules mandate the use of a computer.

The Westgard multirules are designed to be used in a schematic fashion, as shown in Figure 14-10. The quality control result is first assessed using the first rule, or *warning rule*. If this rule is not broken, the next rule is evaluated, and so on. If at any point a rule other than the warning rule is violated, the result is rejected and the method may be considered out of control. Some rules are designed to be used with only one of the two control levels; other rules are designed to be interpreted with the results of both levels.

Warning Rule or 1_{2s} Rule

To interpret the Westgard schematic, the first number in the rule is the number of quality control results that violate the rule. The subscript numbers refer to the Westgard rule that is being violated. The 1_{2s} rule is only a warning rule. This rule is violated if either of the two controls exceeds 2 standard deviations from the mean in either a positive or negative direction. When this rule is violated, the other rules are applied. If the quality control results do not violate any other rule, even if one of the two results violates the 1_{2S} rule, the control results are accepted. This is why the 1_{2S} rule is referred to as the warning rule.

PROBLEM

Below are two Levey-Jennings charts for level I (Figure 14-11A) and level II (Figure 14-11B) glucose control. Note the results obtained for both levels on day 5. Do they violate any Westgard rules?

On day 5, the result for the level I control exceeded +2 standard deviations but was within +3 standard deviations. However, the result for the level II control was within 2 standard deviations. Since only one of the two quality control results exceeded +2 standard deviations, the 1_{2S} warning rule was violated. Since no other rule was violated on that day, the run can be accepted.

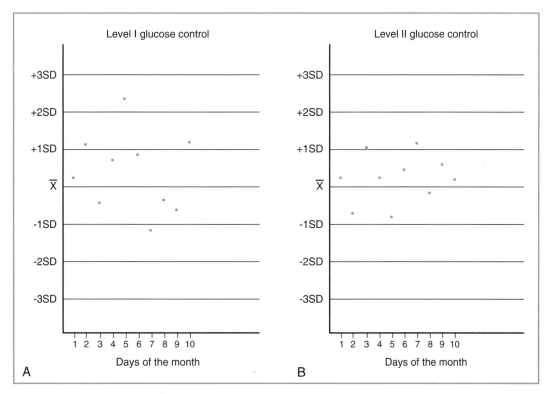

FIGURE 14-11 Levels I (*A*) and II (*B*) glucose controls. (From Doucette, L. J. [1997]. *Mathematics for the Clinical Laboratory* [p. 289]. Philadelphia: W.B. Saunders Company.)

1₃ₛ *Rule*

The 1_{3S} rule is violated when the result of one of the two quality control results is outside of 3 standard deviations. Remember that, statistically, approximately 99% of all results should fall within ±3 standard deviations from the mean. Therefore, if a result is outside of 3 standard deviations, there is less than a 1% chance that it is accurate and a 99.7% chance that it is invalid. Because the chance that a result falls outside of 3 standard deviations is remote (<1%), when either of the quality control results violates this rule, the result is rejected and the run is out of control and cannot be accepted. The 1_{3S} rule is usually violated because of random error. The quality control should be reanalyzed, and if no rules are violated on the repeat analysis, the patient results can be released.

PROBLEM

Below are two Levey-Jennings charts for a level I (Figure 14-12A) and level II (Figure 14-12B) cholesterol control. Note the result for day 7. What rule, if any, is violated?

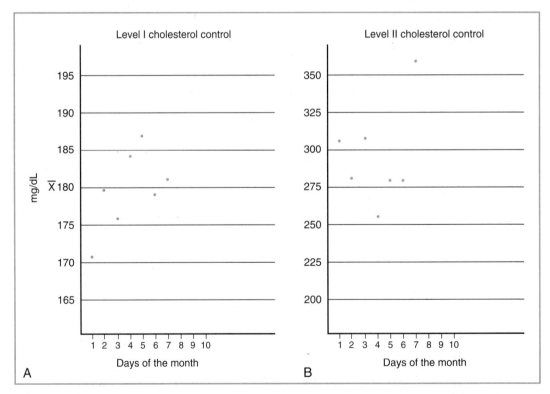

FIGURE 14-12 Levels I (*A*) and II (*B*) cholesterol controls. (From Doucette, L. J. [1997]. *Mathematics for the Clinical Laboratory* [p. 290]. Philadelphia: W.B. Saunders Company.

On day 7, the result for the level II cholesterol control was 360 mg/dL, which exceeded the +3 standard deviation range for this cholesterol control. Note that, by default, if a result exceeds ±3 standard deviations, it violates the 1_{2s} warning rule, thereby setting off the sequential chain of analysis of the rest of the Westgard rules. The next rule to analyze after a result has broken the warning rule is the 1_{3s} rule. The level II cholesterol control has violated this rule. The run cannot be accepted, and the control must be repeated. Usually when a control exceeds 3 standard deviations it is because of a random error and is unlikely to occur again. However, if on repeat analysis the result is still above 3 standard deviations, a different rule that will be discussed next has been violated and the reason is systematic error. Generally, a new bottle of control is used. If that fails to correct the problem, the test method may have to be recalibrated.

2_{2s} Rule

The 2_{2s} rule can be violated in two ways. The first is if both control results are above or below 2 standard deviations from the mean. Both control results must be either above or below 2 standard deviations to violate this rule. The second way this rule can be violated is if one of the control results also exceeded 2 standard deviations in the same manner in the previous run. For example, if one of the control results fell +2.2 standard deviations from the mean for an assay, and the next time the assay was performed the same control fell more than +2 standard deviations again, the 2_{2s} rule has been violated.

PROBLEMS

Below are two quality control charts for level I (Figure 14-13A) and level II (Figure 14-13B) total cholesterol. Notice the quality control results for day 10. Is a Westgard rule violated on that day, and if so, which one?

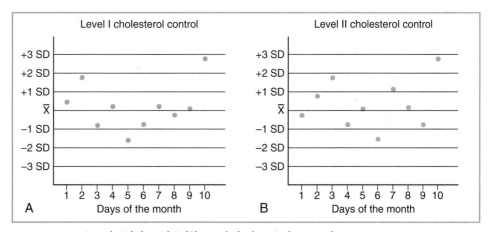

FIGURE 14-13 Levels I (*A*) and II (*B*) total cholesterol controls.

On day 10, both the level I and level II total cholesterol quality control results are more than 2 standard deviations from the mean. Using the Westgard schematic, on day 10 it is noted that the 1_{2s} warning rule is violated for level I (as well as level II). This triggers evaluation of the other rules. The next rule to be evaluated is the 1_{3s} rule. Neither control value violates the 1_{3s} rule. The next rule is the 2_{2s} rule. When this rule is evaluated, it is noted that both control levels exceed +2 standard deviations from the mean, therefore violating the 2_{2s} rule. No other rule is found to be violated. The 2_{2s} rule is violated because of a systematic error in the method. The error must be found and corrected because the method is out of control. No patient results should be reported until the error is corrected and the control results are acceptable.

Below are two quality control charts for level I (Figure 14-14*A*) and level II (Figure 14-14*B*) sodium results. Notice the quality control result on day 4 for level II. Is it in violation of any rule? If so, which one?

On day 4, the level II control exceeded −2 standard deviations from the mean control interval. Thus, the control violated the 1_{2s} warning rule and triggered the evaluation of the other rules. The 1_{3s} rule is not violated, but examination of the previ-

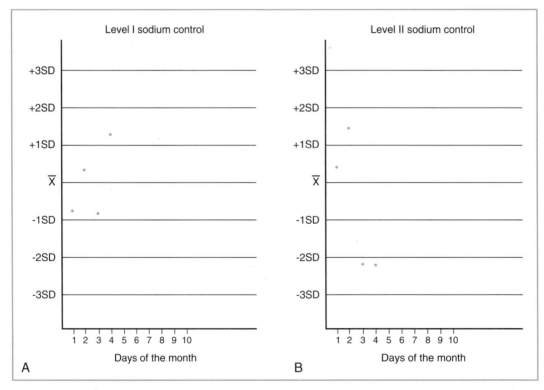

A   B

FIGURE 14-14 Levels I (*A*) and II (*B*) sodium controls. (From Doucette, L. J. [1997]. *Mathematics for the Clinical Laboratory* [p. 292]. Philadelphia: W.B. Saunders Company.)

ous run reveals that the control has violated the 2_{2s} rule. This is because, for two runs in a row, both control results exceeded 2 standard deviations. In this example the control results demonstrate a low bias, but the 2_{2s} rule can also be violated if control results demonstrate a high bias by exceeding the +2 standard deviation interval in a positive rather than a negative direction.

R_{4S} Rule

The R_{4S} rule is violated when the difference, or range, between the two control values within a run is more than 4 standard deviations. For example, if one level of control was −2.2 standard deviations from the mean and the other level of control was +2.0 standard deviations from the mean, the spread of the difference between the two levels is 4.2 standard deviations. Therefore, the R_{4S} rule has been violated. To simplify, the R_{4S} rule is violated when both control values violate the 1_{2S} rule but in opposite directions, that is, one control is above the +2 standard deviation and the other is below the −2 standard deviation. The R_{4S} rule is usually violated because of random error. The run is rejected and patient results are not reported until the method is in control.

PROBLEM

Two levels of quality control for hemoglobin are charted on the Levey-Jennings charts below (Figures 14-15A and 14-15B). Note the control results for day 12. Are any quality control rules violated on that day?

On day 12, the control result for level I was 2.1 standard deviations above the mean. This violated the 1_{2s} rule and triggered review of the other rules. The control result for level II was 2.2 standard deviations below the mean. The spread, or range, between the two control results is 4.3 standard deviations, which violates the R_{4s} rule.

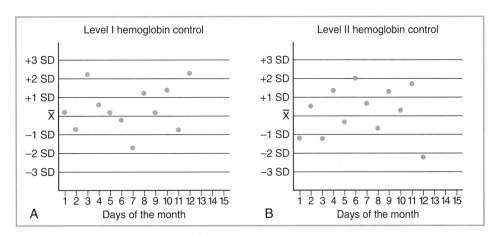

FIGURE 14-15 Levels I (A) and II (B) hemoglobin controls.

4₁s Rule

4₁s Rule

The 4₁s rule can be violated in two ways. The first occurs when one level of control has four consecutive results fall on the same side of the mean and all four exceed +1 or −1 standard deviation of the mean. This rule can also be used with two levels of control. The rule is violated when both levels of control for two runs in a row exceed +1 or −1 standard deviation from the mean. This rule is somewhat like the rule for a shift, that is, the four results are on the same side of the mean (which is statistically unlikely) and exceed 1 standard deviation (but not 2 standard deviations). This rule demonstrates the importance of reviewing not only the immediate quality control results for rule violations but also the previous results.

PROBLEM

Two levels of control for total bilirubin are charted on the Levey-Jennings chart below (Figures 14-16A and 14-16B). Do any of the control results violate any Westgard rules? If so, which one?

On day 4, the level I control violated the 4₁s rule because the control result for that day was the fourth result to fall on the same side of the mean and exceed +1 stan-

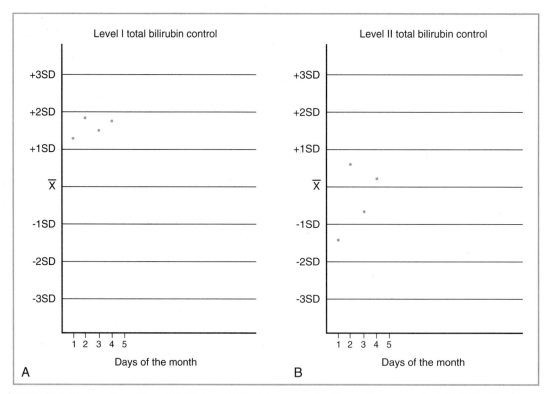

FIGURE 14-16 Levels I (*A*) and II (*B*) total bilirubin controls. (From Doucette, L. J. [1997]. *Mathematics for the Clinical Laboratory* [p. 295]. Philadelphia: W.B. Saunders Company.)

dard deviation from the mean. A systematic error is probably the cause, and the run is rejected until the problem is corrected.

10$_x$ Rule

The 10$_x$ rule can also be violated in two ways. The first is when, for 10 consecutive runs for one level of quality control, the results are all on the same side of the mean. All 10 results can fall above or below the mean. The second way this rule is violated is when the results are all on the same side of the mean for both levels of control for 5 days (or five runs) in a row. The 10$_x$ rule detects shifts and trends and is violated because of systematic error. As with all the other rule violations, patient results are not reported until the method is in control.

PROBLEM

Below are the Levey-Jennings charts (Figures 14-17A and 14-17B) of two levels of control for serum total protein. Do the control results violate any Westgard rules? If so, which one?

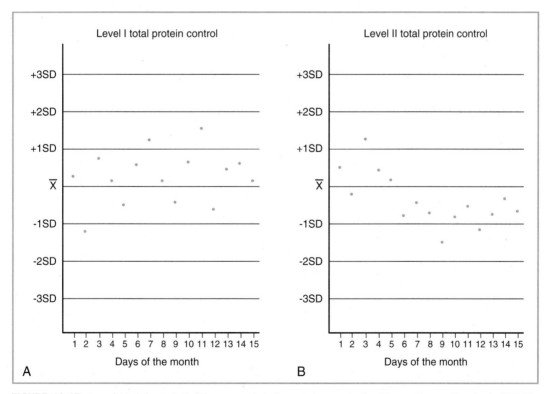

FIGURE 14-17 Levels I (*A*) and II (*B*) serum total protein controls. (From Doucette, L. J. [1997]. *Mathematics for the Clinical Laboratory* [p. 296]. Philadelphia: W.B. Saunders Company.)

The level II control results violate the 10_x rule on day 15. Level I control results do not violate any of the Westgard rules. A systematic error is occurring with the level II control. The patient results cannot be reported until the method is in control.

Westgard Rules for Three Levels of Control

Three levels of control are often used with automated cell counters in the hematology laboratory. As mentioned earlier, three levels of control may also be used for certain chemistry analytes such as therapeutic drugs. The Westgard rules for using three levels of control are similar to those for two levels. Instead of the 2_{2s} rule, the $(2 \text{ of } 3)_{2s}$ rule is used. This rule is violated when two of the three levels of control exceed 2 standard deviations in the same direction. Instead of the 10_x rule, the 9_x rule is used. This rule is violated when nine results in a row for a single control all fall on the same side of the mean or when, for three runs, the results for all three levels of control fall on the same side of the mean. The 4_{1s} rule is not applied when using three levels of control. Figure 14-18 is a control schematic when using three levels of control.

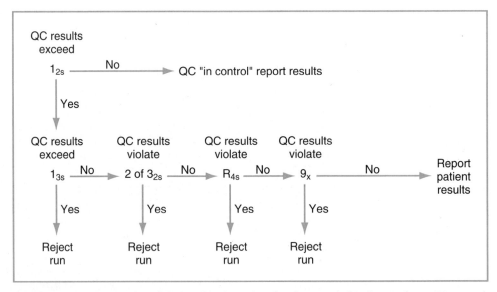

FIGURE 14-18 Westgard multirules for three levels of control. (Redrawn from Westgard, J. O., Barry, P. L., Hunt, M. R., and Groth, T. [1981]. A multi-rule Shewhart chart for quality control in clinical chemistry. *Clinical Chemistry*, 27:493–501.)

EXAMPLE PROBLEMS

This section is designed to be useful to both the student and the health care practitioner. Students can use the example problems in order to master the material. The health care practitioner can use these problems as templates for performing laboratory calculations. Find an example problem similar to the problem that you need to solve and substitute into the equation the numbers appropriate to your calculation.

1. **Q** **The mean for the level I control for a glucose method is 100 mg/dL. One standard deviation is 5 mg/dL. The laboratory uses the ±2 standard deviation range for its criteria for quality control limits. For the first 10 days of the month, the following quality control results (in mg/dL) were obtained (assume that the laboratory operates only one shift): 105, 106, 104, 107, 104, 105, 106, 109, 107, 108. Is anything wrong with the quality control results?**

   A The ±2 standard deviation range for this assay is 90 to 110 mg/dL. All of the quality control results fall within the ±2 standard deviation range. However, these results demonstrate that a shift has occurred, as all of the results are above the mean value of 100 mg/dL and violate the 10_x rule. The cause of the shift must be investigated and corrected.

2. **Q** **A small physician office laboratory uses the ±2 standard deviation cutoff for the quality control limits for its hematology analyzer. The mean for the level II quality control is 8.0×10^9/L and the ±2 standard deviation range is 7.0×10^9/L to 9.0×10^9/L. Ten level I results were obtained on 10 consecutive days. Is there anything wrong with these results? Level I results (in units of 10^9/L) are 7.5, 7.8, 7.9, 8.0, 8.1, 8.3, 8.5, 8.6, 8.7, and 8.8.**

   A None of the results exceed the ±2 standard deviation quality control cutoff limits. However, the results demonstrate an upward trend as they increase in value over time. Quality control results should demonstrate a random pattern of distribution, and these results do not. The cause of the trend must be determined and corrective action taken.

3. **Q** **Using the Westgard multirules criteria and the following quality control results for the level I and level II sodium controls, are the results acceptable? The mean for the level I sodium control is 135**

mmol/L, with a ±2 standard deviation range from 130 to 140 mmol/L. The mean for the level II control is 150 mmol/L, with a ±2 standard deviation range from 145 to 155 mmol/L.

                                  Day

                       1   2   3   4   5   6   7
Level I control results: 135, 136, 131, 135, 136, 138, 133
Level II control results: 144, 145, 150, 152, 149, 150, 148

A On day 1, the level II control exceeded the −2 standard deviation cut-off of 145 mmol/L. However, the level I control fell within acceptable limits. The level II control violated the 1_{2s} rule. This rule is only a warning rule indicating that a problem may be developing. The results are acceptable, and the results of any patient samples run that day can be reported.

4. **Q** Below are Levey-Jennings charts for two levels of control for glucose. Note the results for day 5. Are these results acceptable? If not, what rule is violated?

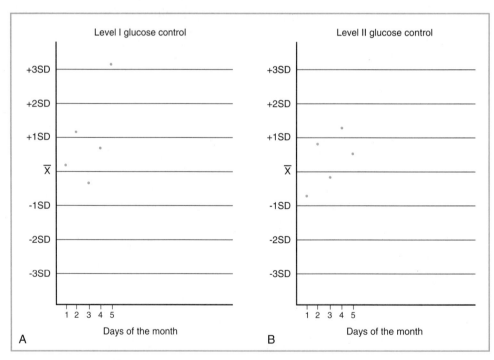

From Doucette, L. J. [1997]. *Mathematics for the Clinical Laboratory* [p. 299]. Philadelphia: W.B. Saunders Company.

A On day 5, the result for the level I glucose control exceeded +3 standard deviations. This violates the 1_{3S} rule. The quality control results cannot be accepted. The cause of the out-of-control results should be investigated.

5. **Q** **Below are the Levey-Jennings charts for level I and level II potassium controls. Are any Westgard rules violated, and if so, which ones?**

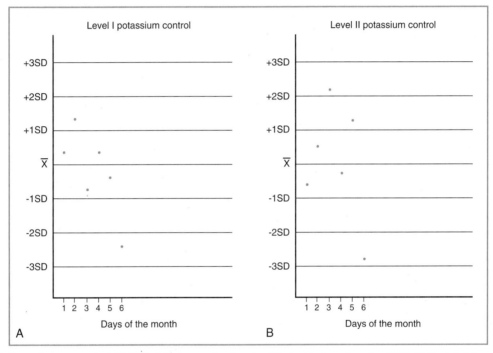

A   B

From Doucette, L. J. [1997]. *Mathematics for the Clinical Laboratory* [p. 300]. Philadelphia: W.B. Saunders Company.

A On day 3, level II violated the 1_{2S} warning rule. Since no other rule was violated, the quality control results were acceptable that day. On day 6, results for both levels of control fell below the 2 standard deviation cutoff but were within 3 standard deviations. This occurrence violates the 2_{2S} rule, which indicates that a systematic problem is affecting the method. The cause of the error must be investigated and corrective action taken.

6. **Q** **On the following page are the Levey-Jennings charts for level I and level II triglyceride controls. Are any Westgard rules violated, and if so, which ones?**

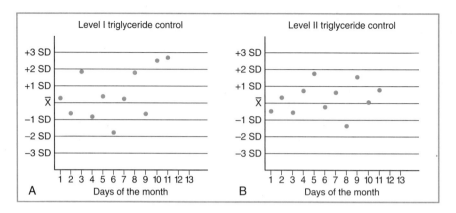

A On day 10, the level I control exceeded +2 standard deviations and therefore violated the 1_{2s} warning rule. However, the level II control for that day did not violate any rules. Thus, the quality control results for that day were acceptable. On day 11, the level I triglyceride control again violated the 1_{2s} rule, as the result again exceeded +2 standard deviations. It also violated the 2_{2s} rule, as two sequential quality control results exceeded 2 standard deviations. Remember that the 2_{2s} rule applies not only to the quality control results for both levels of control measured during a run, but also to one level of control between days. Therefore, it is important to evaluate the control results with respect to prior control results when checking for possible rule violations.

7. **Q** Below are the Levey-Jennings charts for the level I and level II total bilirubin controls. Are any Westgard rules violated, and if so, which ones?

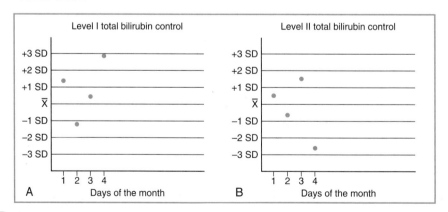

A The R_{4s} rule was violated on day 4 because there is a 4 standard deviation spread between the level I and level II control values. The R_{4s} rule is usually violated because of random error.

8. **Q** Below are two Levey-Jennings charts for level I and level II cholesterol controls. Are any Westgard rules violated, and if so, which ones?

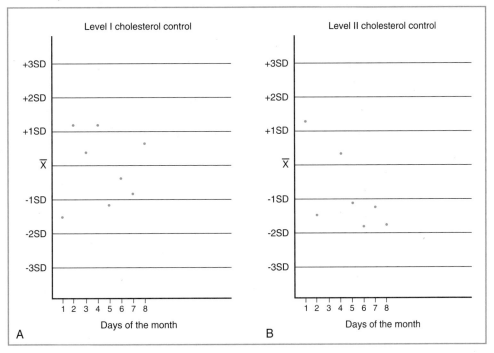

From Doucette, L. J. [1997]. *Mathematics for the Clinical Laboratory* [p. 303]. Philadelphia:
W.B. Saunders Company.

A No rules are violated for the level I control. However, the level II cholesterol control violates the 4_{1s} rule on day 8.

9. **Q** Below are the Levey-Jennings charts for the level I and level II serum potassium controls. Are any Westgard rules violated, and if
so, which ones?

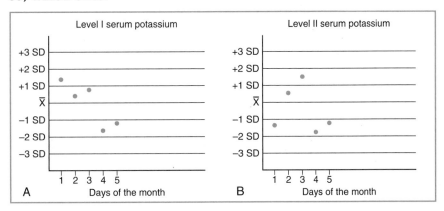

A Note the results on day 5 for both levels of control. On day 5, the 1_{4S} rule was violated because both levels of control exceeded −1 standard deviation for 2 days in a row. This is probably an indication that a shift may be occurring. The method must be investigated to determine the cause of the problem.

10. **Q** Below are the Levey-Jennings charts for level I and level II total protein controls. Are any Westgard rules violated, and if so, which ones?

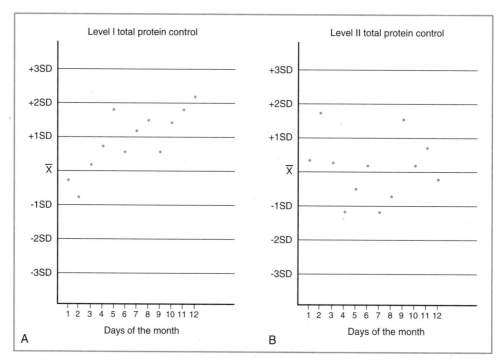

From Doucette, L. J. [1997]. *Mathematics for the Clinical Laboratory* [p. 305]. Philadelphia: W.B. Saunders Company.

A On day 12 for level I the 10_x rule was violated. This rule is violated when, for 10 consecutive runs, the quality control results fall on the same side of the mean. This rule may be violated even if the results do not violate the 1_{2S} or 4_{1S} rule. Statistically, it is highly unlikely that 10 values in a row will fall on the same side of the mean. Rather, there should be random variation, with some results higher and other results lower than the mean. The method should be evaluated to determine the systematic error that is causing the problem.

11. **Q** Below are two Levey-Jennings charts for level I and level II albu-
min controls. Are any Westgard rules violated, and if so, which
ones?

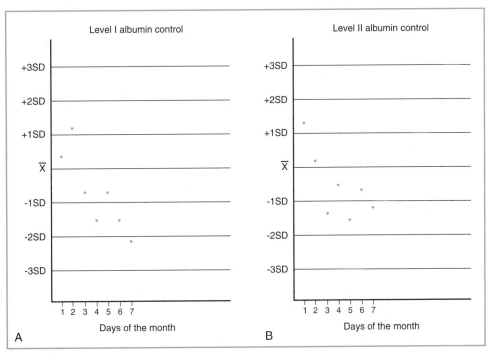

A   B

From Doucette, L. J. [1997]. *Mathematics for the Clinical Laboratory* [p. 306]. W.B. Saunders Company.

A On day 7, the 10_x rule was violated because, for both control levels,
the fifth consecutive control result fell on the same side of the mean.
This is highly unlikely and strongly suggests that a shift is occurring.
The cause of the problem must be investigated.

Practice Problems

Solve the following problems to further master the material. All answers
and explanations to some problems can be found in a separate section at
the back of the book.

1. Describe a shift.
2. Describe a trend.
3. Describe a preanalytical error.

4. Describe an analytical error.
5. Describe a postanalytical error.

Use the Westgard multirules system to answer the following questions.
6. Which rule is the warning rule?
7. What type of error is probably occurring if a 1_{3S} rule violation occurs?
8. What type of error is probably occurring if a 2_{2S} rule violation occurs?
9. How can the R_{4S} rule be violated?
10. How can the 4_{1S} rule be violated?
11. How can the 10_x rule be violated?

REFERENCES

1. U.S. Government. *Title 57, Code of Federal Regulations: Clinical Laboratory Improvement Amendments of 1988: Final Rule.* U.S. Government Printing Office, Washington, DC, February, 1992.
2. Korpman, R. A., and Bull, B. S. The implementation of a robust estimator of the mean for quality control on a programmable calculator or laboratory computer. *American Journal of Clinical Pathology,* 65:252, 1976.
3. Westgard, J. O., Barry P. L., Hunt, M. R., and Groth, T. A multi-rule Shewhart chart for quality control in clinical chemistry. *Clinical Chemistry,* 27:493–501, 1981.
4. Westgard, J. O., Quam, E. F., and Barry, P. L. Selection grids for planning quality control procedures. *Clinical Laboratory Science,* 3:273–280, 1990.

CHAPTER **15**

Instrument and Method Assessment

INTRODUCTION

Determination of the Diagnostic Value of a Method

Diagnostic Sensitivity and Specificity

The goal of the clinical laboratory is to produce accurate and precise results that aid physicians in the diagnosis and treatment of disease states and processes. In addition, the laboratory tests should be able to distinguish between patients who have a disease and those who do not. Figure 15-1 is a graph of two sets of patients tested for a particular disease. The group on the left has the disease; the group on the right does not. The best laboratory test will have no overlap between groups, i.e., a gray area where the physician cannot determine if the patient had the disease. Figure 15-2 demonstrates a test that has an overlap between groups.

Diagnostic *sensitivity* is the probability that only patients with the disease will test positive for the disease. Diagnostic *specificity* is the probability that patients who do not have the disease will test negative for the disease. The best test will have 100% sensitivity and specificity. The best screening test has the highest sensitivity, whereas the best confirmatory test has the highest specificity.

The sensitivity and specificity of a method can be calculated by the following formulas:

$$\text{Sensitivity} = \frac{\text{True positive}}{\text{True positive} + \text{false negative}} \times 100$$

$$\text{Specificity} = \frac{\text{True negative}}{\text{True negative} + \text{false positive}} \times 100$$

where

True positive (TP) = number of individuals who have the disease and test positive

False positive (FP) = number of individuals who do not have the disease but test positive

True negative (TN) = number of individuals who do not have the disease and test negative

False negative (FN) = number of individuals who have the disease but test negative

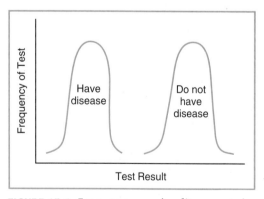

FIGURE 15-1 Frequency graph of two populations showing those who have a particular disease and those who do not have a particular disease.

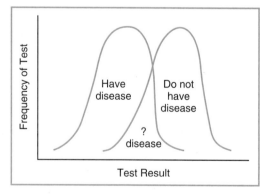

FIGURE 15-2 Frequency graph of two populations with an overlap zone.

PROBLEMS

A new kit was developed to detect the presence of group A streptococcus in throat swabs. The manufacturer tested the kit on 500 pediatric patients with a presumptive diagnosis of group A streptococcus. Three hundred and fifty patients tested positive for group A streptococcus with the kit. Of these 350, 325 were verified by culture to be positive for group A streptococcus. One hundred fifty patients tested negative with the kit; of these, 30 were determined to be positive for group A streptococcus by culture. What is the diagnostic sensitivity and specificity of this new kit?

In order to calculate the diagnostic sensitivity and specificity of this kit, first determine the number of true positive (TP), true negative (TN), false positive (FP), and false negative (FN) test results. If 350 children tested positive by the kit but only 325 of these tests were confirmed, then the number of TPs is 325 and the number of FPs is 25. Since 150 children tested negative by the kit but 30 were actually positive, the number of TNs is 120 and the number of FNs is 30. Therefore, by using the formulas, the diagnostic sensitivity and sensitivity of this kit can be determined.

$$\text{Diagnostic sensitivity} = \frac{325}{325 + 30} \times 100$$

$$= \frac{325}{355} \times 100$$

$$= 91.5\%$$

$$\text{Diagnostic specificity} = \frac{120}{120 + 25} \times 100$$

$$= \frac{120}{145} \times 100$$

$$= 82.8\%$$

Therefore, this new kit is very good at detecting the presence of group A streptococcus in patients infected with the organism but is less effective in determining which children are not infected with the organism.

A new kit was developed to detect qualitative human chorionic gonadotrophin (hCG) in urine. Urine samples from 300 women who were suspected of being pregnant were tested with this new kit. There were 220 positive results and 80 negative results. Of the 220 positive results, 215 were confirmed positive (TP). Of the 80 negative results, 77 were confirmed negative (TN) and 3 were FNs. What is the diagnostic specificity and sensitivity of this new method?

There were 215 TPs, 77 TNs, 5 FPs, and 3 FNs with this method. Therefore:

$$\text{Diagnostic sensitivity} = \frac{215}{215 + 3} \times 100$$

$$= \frac{215}{218} \times 100$$

$$= 98.6\%$$

$$\text{Diagnostic specificity} = \frac{77}{77 + 5} \times 100$$

$$= \frac{77}{82} \times 100$$

$$= 93.9\%$$

Therefore, this new method has high sensitivity and specificity.

Efficiency

In addition to diagnostic sensitivity and specificity, the *efficiency* of the test can be calculated. The efficiency of a test is the number of patients correctly diagnosed as either having or not having the disease, i.e., as TP or TN. The following calculation can be used to determine the efficiency of a laboratory test:

$$\text{Efficiency} = \frac{TP + TN}{TP + FP + FN + TN} \times 100$$

PROBLEMS

Using the data from the first example, what is the efficiency of the new group A streptococcus kit?

Analysis of the new kit revealed:

TP = 325
FP = 25
TN = 120
FN = 30

Using the formula to determine the efficiency of a test, the following equation is derived:

$$\text{Efficiency} = \frac{325 + 120}{325 + 25 + 30 + 120} \times 100$$

$$= \frac{445}{500} \times 100$$

$$= 89.0\%$$

Using the values from the second example concerning an hCG kit, what is this method's efficiency?

$$\text{Efficiency} = \frac{215 + 77}{215 + 5 + 3 + 77} \times 100$$

$$= \frac{292}{300} \times 100$$

$$= 97.3\%$$

Predictive Value

The last statistic that is used to assess the diagnostic value of a test method is *predictive value*. There are two types of predictive value. The first is *positive predictive value*, the ability of a method to determine correctly the presence of a disease in those patients who have the disease. In other words, patients positive for the disease will test positive by the test method. The *negative predictive value* is the ability of a method to determine correctly the absence of a disease in patients who do not have the disease. These patients should test negative by the test method designed to detect the disease.

The positive predictive value is calculated with the following formula:

$$\text{Positive predictive value} = \frac{TP}{TP + FP} \times 100$$

The negative predictive value is calculated with the following formula:

$$\text{Negative predictive value} = \frac{TN}{TN + FN} \times 100$$

PROBLEMS

A new assay was developed to detect prostate cancer prior to the development of clinical symptoms. The manufacturer claimed that the assay was more sensitive and specific than any existing tests for prostate cancer. In a large clinical trial, blood samples from 10,000 men who were asymptomatic for prostate cancer were tested using this new assay. Of this group, 2000 tested positive and 8000 tested negative. Of the 2000 who tested positive, 1900 later developed prostate cancer. Of the 8000 who tested negative, 30 later developed prostate cancer. What is the positive predictive value for this test?

To calculate the positive predictive value, the following formula is used:

$$\text{Positive predictive value} = \frac{TP}{TP + FP} \times 100$$

The number of TPs for this test is 1900, and the number of FPs is 100. Therefore, the positive predictive value is:

$$
\begin{aligned}
\text{Positive predictive value} &= \frac{1900}{1900 + 100} \times 100 \\
&= \frac{1900}{2000} \times 100 \\
&= 95.0\%
\end{aligned}
$$

Using the data from the previous example, what would be the negative predictive value of this new prostate cancer test?

The negative predictive value is calculated by the following formula:

$$\text{Negative predictive value} = \frac{TN}{TN + FN} \times 100$$

Of the 10,000 men tested, 8000 tested negative. However, 30 of these results were FNs, as the men later developed prostate cancer. Therefore, there were 7970 TNs. Using the formula, the negative predictive value is:

$$\text{Negative predictive value} = \frac{7970}{7970 + 30} \times 100$$

$$= \frac{7970}{8000} \times 100$$

$$= 99.6\%$$

Inferential Statistics

Inferential statistics are statistics generally used to compare one or more sets of data to each other for the purpose of inferring certain statistical information. One example is the statistical comparison of the results of two instruments that analyzed the same set of samples to determine if there was a statistically significant difference between the two sets of results. The statistical comparison of methods is a very important quality assurance tool for the laboratory.

Laboratory reports include the normal or *reference* range concentration of every compound analyzed in the laboratory to allow the physician to interpret the result in comparison with the reference range. When a laboratory changes methods or instruments, either because of increased speed and convenience or decreased cost, the result obtained with the new analyzer or method should not differ significantly from the result that would have been obtained with the old analyzer. If the results differ, good laboratory practice and the Clinical Laboratory Improvement Amendment of 1988 (CLIA'88) require the laboratory to establish new reference range concentrations for every compound analyzed with the new instrument or method. How can the laboratory determine if the results obtained with the old analyzer and the new analyzer are the same? A number of inferential statistics can be calculated to answer this question. Most laboratories today use computer programs specifically designed for calculation of these statistics in the clinical laboratory. The information that follows is based on data that are normally distributed and have a sample number or *n* value of at least 30. Information on using more advanced statistics such as population statistics or nonparametric sample distributions can be found in many statistics textbooks.

Student's t-Test

Student's *t*-test is used to determine whether there is a statistical difference (or *bias*) between the means of two methods and can indicate the accuracy of a new method. Student's *t*-test is a statistical test that is not often used in small labora-tories, such as physicians' office laboratories, but it is presented here for those situations in which it may be used, such as when a new instrument is being brought into use and the laboratory wishes to perform its own statistical compari-son rather than depend on the comparison supplied by the vendor. Before the actual calculations are described, some basic information must be given. In gen-eral, one method is considered the reference method and the other method is the test method. Two hypotheses are formed: the null hypothesis (H_0) and the alter-nate hypothesis (H_a). The null hypothesis states that there is no statistically sig-nificant difference between the methods (reference method A is the same as test method B), while the alternate hypothesis states that there is a statistically sig-nificant difference between the methods (reference method A is not the same as test method B). Based on the statistical difference, the null hypothesis is either rejected or accepted. When the null hypothesis is accepted, this decision is de-scribed in statistical terminology as a failure to reject the null hypothesis.

First, determine if you are trying to prove that the results achieved with refer-ence method A are either statistically higher or lower than those achieved with test method B. For example, the null hypothesis may state that "the results with reference method A are higher than those with test method B" or "the results with reference method A are lower than those with test method B." If this is what you are trying to prove, then your *t*-test is called a *one-tailed test*. A one-tailed *t*-test is shown in Figure 15-3. In comparison, a *two-tailed test* has two possible outcomes. Statistically, it may be proven that reference method A is different from test method B. Reference method A may be higher or lower than test method B, as shown in Figure 15-4.

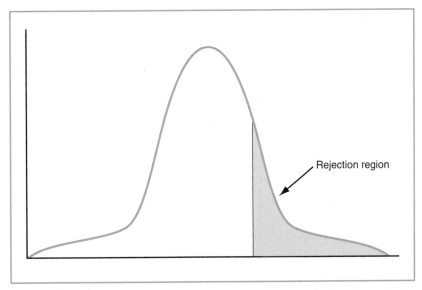

FIGURE 15-3 One-tailed *t*-test. (From Doucette, L. J. [1997]. *Mathematics for the Clinical Laboratory* [p. 317]. Philadelphia: W.B. Saunders Company.)

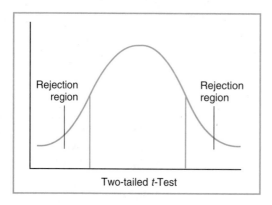

FIGURE 15-4 Two-tailed *t*-test.

Second, you are trying to prove that reference method A is statistically different from test method B. But what does "statistically different" mean? It means that the *t*-test value that you calculate exceeds a mathematical cutoff value and enters what is termed the *critical region,* or rejection region of the *t*-test. Figure 15-5 shows a two-tailed *t*-test with labeled critical and acceptance regions.

Third, you have to decide where that critical region will be. How do you decide this? First, you have to decide what the probability level, or *p*, of rejection will be. That is, how certain do you want to be that you are not rejecting a valid comparison just because, statistically, your results fell outside of a predetermined numerical cutoff value?

This probability level of rejection depends on the degree of certainty, or significance, that is required. Since *p* depends on the significance that is required, it is often referred to as the *significance level.* For example, if a 95% probability level is used for acceptance of the null hypothesis, the significance level of rejection is 5%. The significance level is often expressed as a fraction of 100, i.e., 5% would be expressed as $p = 0.05$ and would indicate the probability of rejection.

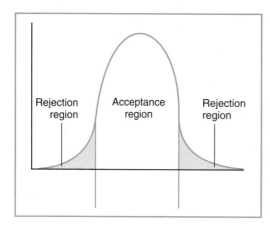

FIGURE 15-5 Two-tailed *t*-test with rejection and acceptance regions.

This $p = 0.05$ would correspond to a numerical cutoff value (the critical region) above which the null hypothesis is rejected or fails to be accepted.

It has been proven statistically that the numerical cutoff point for the 5% confidence limit for a two-tailed test with a sample size of at least 30 is the mean ± 1.96, as shown in Figure 15-6. Note that the 5% significance level is split between both tails of the distribution. Therefore, there is a 2.5% probability that a result will fall into each critical region.

Using $p = 0.05$, if a calculated t value is greater than 1.96, it will fall into the critical region and the null hypothesis will be rejected. If the calculated t value is less than 1.96, then, statistically, there is a failure to reject the null hypothesis and the null hypothesis can be accepted.

The 95% probability level is the most common level used. However, there is a greater degree of certainty if a 99% probability level is used because then there is only a 1% significance level ($p = 0.01$) of the probability of rejection. The probability level that is used will depend on the needs of each laboratory and will determine the statistically obtained values above and below which the null hypothesis is rejected.

The last basic concept to be discussed is *degrees of freedom*. The amount by which any number can vary is dependent on the amount of restriction placed on that number. In a group of 10 numbers ($n = 10$) with a mean of 50, 9 of the numbers have no restrictions. The 10th number is restricted because, based on the values of the previous 9 numbers, the value of the 10th number is fixed. Therefore, the degrees of freedom in this example is 9 or $n - 1$.

A number of formulas are associated with Student's t-test, depending on whether the data are paired or unpaired. For most clinical laboratory applications, the formula for the paired t-test is used. The calculated t value is compared to a value in a t table to determine if it has exceeded the cutoff value. Both the degrees of freedom and the established p value will determine the actual tabulated t value. Further information on the unpaired t-test can be found in statistical textbooks or in *Mathematics for the Clinical Laboratory*, published by W.B. Saunders in 1997.

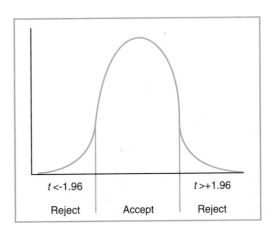

FIGURE 15-6 Two-tailed t-test with $p = 0.05$.

Paired t-Test

The formula for the paired Student's *t*-test is:

$$\text{Paired } t\text{-test} = \frac{[\text{bias}]}{\text{standard deviation of the difference } (s_d) \div \sqrt{n}}$$

where

$$\text{bias } (d) = \text{mean of the differences} = Y_i - X_i$$
$$n = \text{number of paired data}$$
$$s_d = \sqrt{\frac{\Sigma[Y_i - X_i - \text{bias}]^2}{n-1}}$$

PROBLEM

A laboratory wants to purchase a new chemistry analyzer that has a higher throughput than the current analyzer. The laboratory was able to obtain the instrument temporarily to conduct method comparison studies. As part of this study, 20 patient samples were split into two aliquots. Each aliquot was analyzed for glucose on both analyzers. Is there a statistically significant difference (*p* = 0.05) between the results obtained from analyzer A and analyzer B (see Table 15-1)?

To answer this question, it is helpful to phrase it as the null and alternate hypotheses.

H₀ = there is no statistically significant difference between the results obtained with both analyzers

Hₐ = there is a statistically significant difference between the results obtained with both analyzers

To calculate the paired *t*-test value, first obtain the difference between samples (*d*) (see Table 15-2).

Next, subtract the bias from the difference (Y − X) for each pair (see Table 15-3).

Next, to calculate the standard deviation of the difference (Y − X − bias)², square each Y − X − bias value (see Table 15-4).

Next, calculate the standard deviation of the difference:

$$s_d = \sqrt{\frac{\Sigma[Y_i - X_i - \text{bias}]^2}{n-1}}$$

Substituting into the formula the values calculated so far yields:

$$= \sqrt{1869.2 \div 19} = \sqrt{98.38}$$
$$= 9.92$$

Now the paired *t*-test value can be calculated:

$$\text{Paired } t\text{-test} = \frac{\text{bias}}{(s_d) \div \sqrt{n}}$$

TABLE 15-1   Results of Glucose Test with Analyzer A and Analyzer B

Aliquot	Analyzer A (Current Analyzer) (X)	Analyzer B (New Analyzer) (Y)
1	85	86
2	198	195
3	110	113
4	140	142
5	245	210
6	103	99
7	87	78
8	96	99
9	350	359
10	68	64
11	210	215
12	105	103
13	117	112
14	184	193
15	180	168
16	157	153
17	293	287
18	83	81
19	72	79
20	102	112

Substituting the values obtained into the equation yields:

$$\text{Paired } t\text{-test} = \frac{-1.23}{9.92 \div \sqrt{20}}$$

$$= \frac{-1.23}{9.92 \div 4.47}$$

$$= \frac{-1.23}{2.22}$$

$$= -0.554$$

The last step is to determine if the calculated t value exceeds the value obtained from Student's t table in Appendix B. This is a two-tailed test because we are testing to determine if the two methods are different. We are not testing to determine if one method's results are higher or lower than the other. Using Student's t table, find the column under "Area" in the two tails at the $p = 0.05$ significance level. Since we have 20 samples, the number of degrees of freedom is 19. Next, find the number 19 under the column "df" (degrees of freedom). Look across the row until it intersects the 0.05 significance column. The number 2.093 is our tabulated t value. Our calculated t value is -0.554. Any calculated t value greater than 2.045 would

TABLE 15-2 Difference between Samples (d)

Aliquot	Analyzer A (X)	Analyzer B (Y)	d (Y − X)
1	85	86	1
2	198	195	−3
3	110	113	3
4	140	142	2
5	245	210	−35
6	103	99	−4
7	87	78	−9
8	96	99	3
9	350	359	9
10	68	64	−4
11	210	215	5
12	105	103	−2
13	117	112	−5
14	184	193	9
15	180	168	−12
16	157	153	−4
17	293	287	−6
18	83	81	−2
19	72	79	7
20	102	112	10

$$\Sigma = 1 + (-3) + 3 + 2 + (-35) \cdots +10 = -37$$

bias $(d) = \dfrac{-37}{30}$

bias $(d) = -1.23$

fall into the rejection portion of the t distribution. Since −0.554 is less than 2.045, we fail to reject the null hypothesis, i.e., we accept the null hypothesis. Therefore, there is no statistical difference between the glucose results obtained on the new and old analyzers.

F-Test

A very simple statistical test is the F-test. This test is used to compare the precision of two analytical methods. Like Student's t-test, the F-test has an associated probability table for assessment of the calculated F-value. However, unlike Student's t-test, there are separate F probability tables for each probability. Appendix C contains an F probability table for $p = 0.05$. The formula for the F value uses the variances of the methods for comparison (see Chapter 13 for a review of calculation of variance) and is calculated as follows:

TABLE 15-3 Obtaining Y − X − Bias Values

Aliquot	Analyzer A (X)	Analyzer B (Y)	(Y − X)	(Y − X − bias)
1	85	86	1	−0.23
2	198	195	−3	−1.77
3	110	113	3	4.23
4	140	142	2	3.23
5	245	210	−35	−33.77
6	103	99	−4	−2.77
7	87	78	−9	−7.77
8	96	99	3	4.23
9	350	359	9	10.23
10	68	64	−4	−2.77
11	210	215	5	6.23
12	105	103	−2	−0.77
13	117	112	−5	−3.77
14	184	193	9	10.23
15	180	168	−12	−10.77
16	157	153	−4	−2.77
17	293	287	−6	−4.77
18	83	81	−2	−0.77
19	72	79	7	8.23
20	102	112	10	11.23

$$\text{Calculated } F \text{ value} = \frac{\text{larger variance}}{\text{smaller variance}} \quad \text{or} \quad \frac{(\text{standard deviation})^2}{(\text{standard deviation})^2}$$

Once the F value has been calculated, it must be compared to the appropriate F score from the F table. The tabulated F score is dependent on the degrees of freedom for each of the two measurements. Degrees of freedom for each method are calculated by $n − 1$.

PROBLEM

Hemoglobin values obtained by two hematology analyzers were compared. The level I control was analyzed 30 times on each analyzer. The mean, standard deviation, and coefficient of variation for each analyzer were calculated. The standard deviation of analyzer A was 2.1, and that of analyzer B was 1.8. Using the F-test, determine if there is a statistical difference between the precision of analyzer B and analyzer A.

The formula for the F-test is:

$$\text{Calculated } F \text{ value} = \frac{\text{Larger variance}}{\text{Smaller variance}}$$

TABLE 15-4 Determining the Standard Deviation of the Difference

Aliquot	Analyzer A (X)	Analyzer B (Y)	$(Y - X)$	$(Y - X - bias)$	$(Y - X - bias)^2$
1	85	86	1	-0.23	0.05
2	198	195	-3	-1.77	3.13
3	110	113	3	4.23	17.89
4	140	142	2	3.23	10.4
5	245	210	-35	-33.77	1140.41
6	103	99	-4	-2.77	7.67
7	87	78	-9	-7.77	60.37
8	96	99	3	4.23	17.89
9	350	359	9	10.23	104.65
10	68	64	-4	-2.77	7.67
11	210	215	5	6.23	38.81
12	105	103	-2	-0.77	0.59
13	117	112	-5	-3.77	14.21
14	184	193	9	10.23	104.65
15	180	168	-12	-10.77	115.99
16	157	153	-4	-2.77	7.67
17	293	287	-6	-4.77	22.75
18	83	81	-2	-0.77	0.59
19	72	79	7	8.23	67.7
20	102	112	10	11.23	126.11
					$\Sigma = 1869.2$

The standard deviation (SD) is the square root of the variance. By squaring each standard deviation value, the variance for each method can be determined.

Analyzer A: SD of 2.1 $(2.1)^2$ = variance of 4.41
Analyzer B: SD of 1.8 $(1.8)^2$ = variance of 3.24

$$\text{Calculated } F \text{ value} = \frac{4.41}{3.24}$$

Calculated F value = 1.36

Next, the calculated F value is compared to the tabulated F value obtained from Appendix C. With each method, $n = 30$; therefore, each method's degree of freedom is 29. To use the F table, since there are 29 degrees of freedom for analyzer A, use the column with the heading 24. Find the number 29 in the column marked "n_2." The number at the intersection of both columns is 1.90. This is the F cutoff value. The calculated F value is 1.36, which is lower than the cutoff value. Therefore, we fail to reject H_0 and there is no statistical difference in precision between the two analyzers.

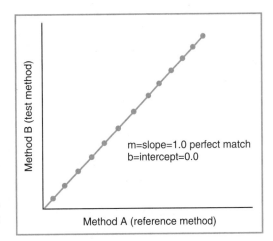

FIGURE 15-7 Linear regression demonstrating perfect correlation between methods.

Linear Regression Analysis by the Method of Least Squares

Student's *t*-test and the *F*-test are useful but limited statistical tools when comparing methods. Both may indicate that there is indeed a statistical difference between methods, but neither can give information on the cause of the difference. One statistical tool often used in the clinical laboratory for method comparison is linear regression analysis. As with Student's *t*-test, the traditional method is considered the reference method, and the new method is considered the test method. In linear regression analysis, samples are tested by both methods. Then the results obtained with each method are plotted on linear graph paper. The results of the reference method are plotted on the *x*-axis, and the results of the test method are plotted on the *y*-axis. If, for each sample tested, the results for both test and reference method are identical, there is perfect correlation between the methods and a perfectly linear line, as demonstrated in Figure 15-7.

A fuller discussion of how to calculate linear regression is beyond the scope of this textbook. Further information on linear regression analysis can be found in many statistical textbooks, including *Mathematics for the Clinical Laboratory*, published by W.B. Saunders in 1997.

Proficiency Testing

Proficiency testing (PT) is a quality assurance tool used to assess the accuracy and precision of the laboratory's methods and instruments. CLIA'88 has mandated the use of PT three times a year for all laboratories performing moderate- or high-complexity tests. In addition, although not mandated legally, many manufacturers of waived tests recommend PT as good laboratory practice. Many organizations and companies supply laboratories with PT samples. Each PT consists of five samples that must be analyzed in the same manner as patient samples. The laboratory analyzes the samples, records the results on the supplied form, and sends the results to the PT agency.

The PT agency then analyzes the data for each analyte and uses many different methods to determine the range of acceptable answers. Many analytes are divided into peer groups based on the method and instrument used for analysis. In this method, a standard deviation index (SDI) is calculated from a peer group standard deviation. The SDI is calculated using the following formula:

$$\text{SDI} = \frac{\text{result from lab} - \text{peer group result}}{\text{standard deviation of peer group}}$$

Sometimes the number of participants using a particular method may not be large enough to allow the SDI to be used for evaluative purposes. The PT agency may then place them in a similar group or use another method of evaluation, the comparative method, for analysis.

In the comparative method, the results obtained with peer groups are compared to those obtained with a historically acceptable method. The comparative method is also used to evaluate results submitted from laboratories that cannot participate in peer group evaluation because they do not have enough peer group members.

Another method is the fixed limits method. Some analytes have a target value that is determined either by the comparative method or by the peer group. The target value will have a small (fixed) variable range. Appendix D lists the acceptable ranges established by the U.S. Health Care Financing Administration (HCFA) for many analytes. Each sample is scored as acceptable or unacceptable, depending on whether it falls inside or outside of the acceptable range.

A few months after the PT results have been submitted to the agency, the agency will send each participating laboratory a summary report. On this report will be the PT score for each analyte. Since each proficiency test event includes five samples to be tested for each analyte, for most analytes four of the five samples (80%) must be scored as acceptable for the laboratory to achieve a passing, or "Satisfactory," score for that analyte. For some analytes, such as immunohematology analytes, a score of 100% must be obtained.

Also on this summary report will be the mean and standard deviation obtained for each analyte, as well as the CV. This information can be used by every laboratory to compare the precision of its instrumentation to that of its peer group.

PT is an important tool that HCFA utilizes to assess the quality of each laboratory. If a laboratory fails to achieve a passing score on an analyte for a single event, the laboratory must investigate the cause of failure, correct it, and document the corrective action. If a laboratory fails to achieve a passing score on an analyte for two consecutive events or two of three testing events, it must contact its PT agency as well as its accreditation agency (e.g., COLA, Joint Commission on the Accreditation of Healthcare Organizations [JCAHO], HCFA, College of American Pathologists [CAP]).

If a laboratory repeatedly fails PT events, it may be asked to stop testing for that analyte by either its PT agency or its accreditation agency. Failure by a laboratory to comply with efforts to improve the quality of its testing, as measured by PT analysis, may result in HCFA revoking the laboratory's CLIA license and putting it out of business.

EXAMPLE PROBLEMS

This section is designed to be useful to both the student and the health care practitioner. Students can use the example problems in order to master the material. The health care practitioner can use these problems as templates for solving laboratory calculations. Find an example problem similar to the problem that you need to solve and substitute into the equation the numbers appropriate to your calculation.

Use the following situation to answer example problems 1–5.
Situation: A new urine pregnancy test kit was developed and tested on 400 women attending an obstetric-gynecology clinic. A total of 160 women tested positive. Of these, 148 pregnancies were confirmed by other means. Of the remaining 240 women who tested negative, 5 were confirmed to be pregnant by other means.

1. **Q** **What is the diagnostic sensitivity of this new assay?**

   A Diagnostic sensitivity is calculated by the following formula:

   $$\text{Sensitivity} = \frac{TP}{TP + FN} \times 100$$

   The number of TPs is 148, and the number of FNs is 5.
   Therefore, the diagnostic sensitivity of this kit is:

   $$\text{Sensitivity} = \frac{148}{148 + 5} \times 100$$

   $$= \frac{148}{153} \times 100$$

   $$= 96.7 \times 100$$

   $$= 96.7\%.$$

2. **Q** **What is the diagnostic specificity of the new pregnancy kit?**

   A The formula for diagnostic specificity is as follows:

   $$\text{Specificity} = \frac{TN}{TN + FP} \times 100$$

The number of TNs is 235, and the number of FPs is 12. Therefore, the diagnostic specificity of this kit is:

$$\text{Specificity} = \frac{235}{235 + 12} \times 100$$

$$= \frac{235}{247} \times 100$$

$$= 0.951 \times 100$$

$$= 95.1\%.$$

3. Q What is the efficiency of this new pregnancy kit?

A The efficiency of a test is measured by the number of patients correctly diagnosed as having or not having the disease or condition. The formula for efficiency is:

$$\text{Efficiency} = \frac{\text{TP} + \text{TN}}{\text{TP} + \text{FP} + \text{FN} + \text{TN}} \times 100$$

$$\text{TP} = 148 \qquad \text{FP} = 12$$
$$\text{TN} = 235 \qquad \text{FN} = 5$$

Substituting into the formula the obtained values yields:

$$\text{Efficiency} = \frac{148 + 235}{148 + 12 + 5 + 235} \times 100$$

$$= \frac{383}{400} \times 100$$

$$= 0.958 \times 100$$

$$= 95.8\%.$$

4. Q What is the positive predictive value of this new pregnancy kit?

A The positive predictive value is the ability of the test to determine correctly the presence of a disease or condition in those patients who have the disease or condition. It is calculated by the following formula:

$$\text{Positive predictive value} = \frac{\text{TP}}{\text{TP} + \text{FP}} \times 100$$

Therefore, the positive predictive value of this new kit is:

$$\text{Positive predictive value} = \frac{148}{148 + 12} \times 100$$

$$= \frac{148}{160} \times 100$$

$$= 0.925 \times 100$$

$$= 92.5\%.$$

5. **Q** **What is the negative predictive value of this new pregnancy kit?**

   A The negative predictive value is the ability of the test to determine correctly the absence of the disease or condition in patients who do not have the disease or condition. The negative predictive value is calculated by the following formula:

$$\text{Negative predictive value} = \frac{TN}{TN + FN} \times 100$$

   Since there were 235 TNs and 5 FNs, the negative predictive value of this kit is:

$$\begin{aligned} \text{Negative predictive value} &= \frac{235}{235 + 5} \times 100 \\ &= \frac{235}{240} \times 100 \\ &= 0.979 \times 100 \\ &= 97.9\%. \end{aligned}$$

6. **Q** **What is the null hypothesis and the alternate hypothesis in inferential statistics?**

   A Inferential statistics are statistics used to compare groups of data to determine if there are significant differences between them. The null hypothesis (H_0) states that there is no statistically significant difference between the groups of data. The alternate hypothesis (H_a) states that there is a statistically significant difference between the two data groups.

7. **Q** **What is Student's *t*-test?**

   A Student's *t*-test is used in the clinical laboratory to compare the means of two methods. The test can detect bias between the methods (i.e., one method yields higher or lower values than the other).

8. **Q** **What is the difference between a one- and a two-tailed Student's *t*-test?**

   A A one-tailed Student's *t*-test is used when one method is tested to determine if it yields data that are greater or less than the data produced by the other method. For example, the laboratory may only be interested in determining if the test method yields higher values than the reference method. In contrast, a two-tailed Student's *t*-test determines if there is a difference, either higher or lower in value, between the methods.

9. **Q** **What are degrees of freedom?**

   A The degrees of freedom used in statistical analyses represent the amount by which any number can vary within a group of numbers. The amount by which any number can vary depends on the restrictions placed on that number. In general, degrees of freedom are calculated by the total number of data points minus 1, i.e., $n - 1$.

10. **Q** **A laboratory received a new hematology analyzer. Before putting it into service, the supervisor analyzed the total white blood count using a normal control 30 times on each analyzer. If the difference between samples, or bias (d), is 3.8 and the standard deviation of the differences (s_d) is 7.83, calculate the paired t value and determine if there is a statistically significant difference at $p < 0.05$.**

   A The paired Student's t-test is calculated by the following formula:

   $$\frac{\text{bias}}{\text{standard deviation of the difference } (s_d) \div \sqrt{n}}$$

   Substituting into the formula the values from the problem yields:

   $$\text{Paired } t\text{-test value} = \frac{3.83}{7.83 \div \sqrt{30}}$$

   $$= \frac{3.83}{7.83} \div 5.48$$

   $$= \frac{3.83}{1.43}$$

   $$= 2.678$$

   The two-tailed Student's t table in Appendix B can be used to determine if the calculated t value is statistically significant. The significance level is 0.05, and since there were 30 values, the degrees of freedom is 29 ($n - 1$). The tabulated value is 2.045. Since the calculated value is larger than the tabulated value, the null hypothesis cannot be accepted. Therefore, there is a statistically significant difference (at $p < 0.05$) between the two hematology analyzers for total white blood cell counts.

11. **Q** **Two coagulation analyzers were compared for precision analysis. The same control was used to analyze 30 replicate prothrombin times on both analyzers. The mean, standard deviation, and CV were determined for the data generated from each analyzer. The standard deviation of analyzer A was 2.1, and the standard deviation of analyzer B was 1.9. Using the F-test, determine if there is a statistically significant difference (at $p < 0.05$) between the precision of analyzers A and B.**

A The F-test is the ratio of the larger variance divided by the smaller variance between two methods. The variance is the square of the standard deviation value. Therefore, the variance of each analyzer is:

Analyzer A   SD = 2.1, variance = $(2.1)^2$ = 4.41
Analyzer B   SD = 1.9, variance = $(1.9)^2$ = 3.61

$$F \text{ value} = \frac{\text{larger variance}}{\text{smaller variance}} = \frac{4.41}{3.61}$$
$$= 1.22.$$

Next, use the F table in Appendix C. Each method has an n of 30; therefore, each analyzer has a degree of freedom value of 29. From the F table, the critical value is 1.90. Since the calculated value is less than the tabulated value, the conclusion is that there is no significant difference in the precision of the two analyzers.

PRACTICE PROBLEMS

Solve the following problems to further master the material. All answers and explanations to some problems can be found in a separate section at the back of the book.

Given the following information for a new diagnostic test, answer questions 1–5. From an evaluative study of 1000 persons the following statistics were generated: TP = 800, TN = 160, FP = 25, and FN = 15.

1. What is the diagnostic sensitivity of the new test?
2. What is the diagnostic specificity of the new test?
3. What is the efficiency of the new test?
4. What is the positive predictive value of the new test?
5. What is the negative predictive value of the new test?
6. A new analyzer was evaluated to replace the laboratory's older analyzer. Twenty samples were tested on each analyzer. The calculated bias was −1.5, and the standard deviation of the difference (s_d) was 12.5. If $p = 0.5$, calculate the t-test value and determine if there is a statistically significant difference between the results obtained with the old and new analyzers.
7. Given the variance of method A, 3.7 ($n = 50$), and the variance of method B, 4.2 ($n = 50$), is there a statistically significant difference ($p < 0.5$) in precision between the two methods?

Preparing a 0.5 McFarland Standard Suspension

1. Add 0.5 mL of 0.048 M $BaCl_2$ (1.175% $BaCl_2 \cdot 2H_2O$ w/v) to 99.5 mL of 0.18 M H_2SO_4 (1% w/v).

2. Mix well with a magnetic stirrer.

3. Distribute 1–5 mL of the resulting standard into screw-cap tubes of the same size used in growing the broth culture inoculum. The amount placed in each tube should be the same as that used in the tests.

4. Seal the tubes tightly with Parafilm.

5. Store in the dark at room temperature.

6. Before use, *vigorously agitate the standard suspension on a mechanical vortex.*

Note: Cultures adjusted to this standard suspension contain approximately 10^8 CFU/mL.

Student *t* Table

This table gives percentage points of the *t* distribution (the values of *t* for differing df that cut off specified proportions of the area in one and in two tails of the *t* distribution).

	Area in Two Tails				
	.10	**.05**	**.02** Area in One Tail	**.01**	**.001**
df	**.05**	**.025**	**.01**	**.005**	**.0005**
1	6.314	12.706	31.821	63.657	636.619
2	2.920	4.303	6.965	9.925	31.598
3	2.353	3.182	4.541	5.841	12.941
4	2.132	2.776	3.747	4.604	8.610
5	2.015	2.571	3.365	4.032	6.859
6	1.943	2.447	3.143	3.707	5.959
7	1.895	2.365	2.998	3.499	5.405
8	1.860	2.306	2.896	3.355	5.041
9	1.833	2.262	2.821	3.250	4.781
10	1.812	2.228	2.764	3.169	4.587
11	1.796	2.201	2.718	3.106	4.437
12	1.782	2.179	2.681	3.055	4.318
13	1.771	2.160	2.650	3.012	4.221
14	1.761	2.145	2.624	2.977	4.140
15	1.753	2.131	2.602	2.947	4.073
16	1.746	2.120	2.583	2.921	4.015
17	1.740	2.110	2.567	2.898	3.965
18	1.734	2.101	2.552	2.878	3.922
19	1.729	2.093	2.539	2.861	3.883
20	1.725	2.086	2.528	2.845	3.850

Continued

APPENDIX B *Continued*

df	Area in Two Tails				
	.10	.05	.02	.01	.001
			Area in One Tail		
	.05	.025	.01	.005	.0005
21	1.721	2.080	2.518	2.831	3.819
22	1.717	2.074	2.508	2.819	3.792
23	1.714	2.069	2.500	2.807	3.767
24	1.711	2.064	2.492	2.797	3.745
25	1.708	2.060	2.485	2.787	3.725
26	1.706	2.056	2.479	2.779	3.707
27	1.703	2.052	2.473	2.771	3.690
28	1.701	2.048	2.467	2.763	3.674
29	1.699	2.045	2.462	2.756	3.659
30	1.697	2.042	2.457	2.750	3.646
40	1.684	2.021	2.423	2.704	3.551
60	1.671	2.000	2.390	2.660	3.460
120	1.658	1.980	2.358	2.617	3.373
∞	1.645	1.960	2.326	2.576	3.291

Data from Table 12: Percentage points of the t-distribution, p. 146 in Biometrika Tables for Statisticians, Vol. 1, 3rd ed., 1966, by E. S. Pearson and H. O. Hartley.

F Probability Table

Denominator Degrees of Freedom	$F_{.95}$								
	Numerator Degrees of Freedom								
	1	**2**	**3**	**4**	**5**	**6**	**7**	**8**	**9**
1	161.4	199.5	215.7	224.6	230.2	234.0	236.8	238.9	240.5
2	18.51	19.00	19.16	19.25	19.30	19.33	19.35	19.37	19.38
3	10.13	9.55	9.28	9.12	9.01	8.94	8.89	8.85	8.81
4	7.71	6.94	6.59	6.39	6.26	6.16	6.09	6.04	6.00
5	6.61	5.79	5.41	5.19	5.05	4.95	4.88	4.82	4.77
6	5.99	5.14	4.76	4.53	4.39	4.28	4.21	4.15	4.10
7	5.59	4.74	4.35	4.12	3.97	3.87	3.79	3.73	3.68
8	5.32	4.46	4.07	3.84	3.69	3.58	3.50	3.44	3.39
9	5.12	4.26	3.86	3.63	3.48	3.37	3.29	3.23	3.18
10	4.96	4.10	3.71	3.48	3.33	3.22	3.14	3.07	3.02
11	4.84	3.98	3.59	3.36	3.20	3.09	3.01	2.95	2.90
12	4.75	3.89	3.49	3.26	3.11	3.00	2.91	2.85	2.80
13	4.67	3.81	3.41	3.18	3.03	2.92	2.83	2.77	2.71
14	4.60	3.74	3.34	3.11	2.96	2.85	2.76	2.70	2.65
15	4.54	3.68	3.29	3.06	2.90	2.79	2.71	2.64	2.59
16	4.49	3.63	3.24	3.01	2.85	2.74	2.66	2.59	2.54
17	4.45	3.59	3.20	2.96	2.81	2.70	2.61	2.55	2.49
18	4.41	3.55	3.16	2.93	2.77	2.66	2.58	2.51	2.46
19	4.38	3.52	3.13	2.90	2.74	2.63	2.54	2.48	2.42
20	4.35	3.49	3.10	2.87	2.71	2.60	2.51	2.45	2.39
21	4.32	3.47	3.07	2.84	2.68	2.57	2.49	2.42	2.37
22	4.30	3.44	3.05	2.82	2.66	2.55	2.46	2.40	2.34
23	4.28	3.42	3.03	2.80	2.64	2.53	2.44	2.37	2.32
24	4.26	3.40	3.01	2.78	2.62	2.51	2.42	2.36	2.30

Continued

APPENDIX C *Continued*

$F_{.95}$

Denominator Degrees of Freedom	Numerator Degrees of Freedom								
	1	**2**	**3**	**4**	**5**	**6**	**7**	**8**	**9**
25	4.24	3.39	2.99	2.76	2.60	2.49	2.40	2.34	2.28
26	4.23	3.37	2.98	2.74	2.59	2.47	2.39	2.32	2.27
27	4.21	3.35	2.96	2.73	2.57	2.46	2.37	2.31	2.25
28	4.20	3.34	2.95	2.71	2.56	2.45	2.36	2.29	2.24
29	4.18	3.33	2.93	2.70	2.55	2.43	2.35	2.28	2.22
30	4.17	3.32	2.92	2.69	2.53	2.42	2.33	2.27	2.21
40	4.08	3.23	2.84	2.61	2.45	2.34	2.25	2.18	2.12
60	4.00	3.15	2.76	2.53	2.37	2.25	2.17	2.10	2.04
120	3.92	3.07	2.68	2.45	2.29	2.17	2.09	2.02	1.96
∞	3.84	3.00	2.60	2.37	2.21	2.10	2.01	1.94	1.88

Denominator Degrees of Freedom	Numerator Degrees of Freedom									
	10	**12**	**15**	**20**	**24**	**30**	**40**	**60**	**120**	**∞**
1	241.9	243.9	245.9	248.0	249.1	250.1	251.1	252.2	253.3	254.3
2	19.40	19.41	19.43	19.45	19.45	19.46	19.47	19.48	19.49	19.50
3	8.79	8.74	8.70	8.66	8.64	8.62	8.59	8.57	8.55	8.53
4	5.96	5.91	5.86	5.80	5.77	5.75	5.72	5.69	5.66	5.63
5	4.74	4.68	4.62	4.56	4.53	4.50	4.46	4.43	4.40	4.36
6	4.06	4.00	3.94	3.87	3.84	3.81	3.77	3.74	3.70	3.67
7	3.64	3.57	3.51	3.44	3.41	3.38	3.34	3.30	3.27	3.23
8	3.35	3.28	3.22	3.15	3.12	3.08	3.04	3.01	2.97	2.93
9	3.14	3.07	3.01	2.94	2.90	2.86	2.83	2.79	2.75	2.71
10	2.98	2.91	2.85	2.77	2.74	2.70	2.66	2.62	2.58	2.54
11	2.85	2.79	2.72	2.65	2.61	2.57	2.53	2.49	2.45	2.40
12	2.75	2.69	2.62	2.54	2.51	2.47	2.43	2.38	2.34	2.30
13	2.67	2.60	2.53	2.46	2.42	2.38	2.34	2.30	2.25	2.21
14	2.60	2.53	2.46	2.39	2.35	2.31	2.27	2.22	2.18	2.13
15	2.54	2.48	2.40	2.33	2.29	2.25	2.20	2.16	2.11	2.07
16	2.49	2.42	2.35	2.28	2.24	2.19	2.15	2.11	2.06	2.01
17	2.45	2.38	2.31	2.23	2.19	2.15	2.10	2.06	2.01	1.96
18	2.41	2.34	2.27	2.19	2.15	2.11	2.06	2.02	1.97	1.92
19	2.38	2.31	2.23	2.16	2.11	2.07	2.03	1.98	1.93	1.88
20	2.35	2.28	2.20	2.12	2.08	2.04	1.99	1.95	1.90	1.84
21	2.32	2.25	2.18	2.10	2.05	2.01	1.96	1.92	1.87	1.81
22	2.30	2.23	2.15	2.07	2.03	1.98	1.94	1.89	1.84	1.78

Table continued on following page

APPENDIX C *Continued*

Denominator Degrees of Freedom	Numerator Degrees of Freedom									
	10	**12**	**15**	**20**	**24**	**30**	**40**	**60**	**120**	**∞**
23	2.27	2.20	2.13	2.05	2.01	1.96	1.91	1.86	1.81	1.76
24	2.25	2.18	2.11	2.03	1.98	1.94	1.89	1.84	1.79	1.73
25	2.24	2.16	2.09	2.01	1.96	1.92	1.87	1.82	1.77	1.71
26	2.22	2.15	2.07	1.99	1.95	1.90	1.85	1.80	1.75	1.69
27	2.20	2.13	2.06	1.97	1.93	1.88	1.84	1.79	1.73	1.67
28	2.19	2.12	2.04	1.96	1.91	1.87	1.82	1.77	1.71	1.65
29	2.18	2.10	2.03	1.94	1.90	1.85	1.81	1.75	1.70	1.64
30	2.16	2.09	2.01	1.93	1.89	1.84	1.79	1.74	1.68	1.62
40	2.08	2.00	1.92	1.84	1.79	1.74	1.69	1.64	1.58	1.51
60	1.99	1.92	1.84	1.75	1.70	1.65	1.59	1.53	1.47	1.39
120	1.91	1.83	1.75	1.66	1.61	1.55	1.50	1.43	1.35	1.25
∞	1.83	1.75	1.67	1.57	1.52	1.46	1.39	1.32	1.22	1.00

Data from Daniel, W. W.: Biostatistics: A Foundation for Analysis in the Health Sciences. New York, John Wiley & Sons, Inc., 1978. Copyright 1978.

CLIA '88 Criteria for Acceptable Performance

Analyte or Test	Criteria for Acceptable Performance
Immunology Laboratory	
Alpha-1 antitrypsin	Target value +/− 3 SD
Alpha fetoprotein (tumor marker)	Target value +/− 3 SD
Antinuclear antibodies	Target value +/− 2 dilutions or positive or negative
Antistreptolysin O	Target value +/− 2 dilutions or positive or negative
Antihuman immunodeficiency virus	Reactive or nonreactive
Complement C3	Target value +/− 3 SD
Complement C4	Target value +/− 3 SD
Hepatitis (HBsAg, HBc, HBeAg)	Reactive or nonreactive
IgA	Target value +/− 3 SD
IgE	Target value +/− 3 SD
IgG	Target value +/− 25%
IgM	Target value +/− 3 SD
Infectious mononucleosis	Target value +/− 2 dilutions or positive or negative
Rheumatoid fever	Target value +/− 2 dilutions or positive or negative
Rubella	Target value +/− 2 dilutions or immune or nonimmune or positive or negative
Chemistry Laboratory	
ALT	Target value +/− 20%
Albumin	Target value +/− 10%
Alkaline phosphatase	Target value +/− 30%
Amylase	Target value +/− 30%
AST	Target value +/− 20%

Table continued on following page

APPENDIX D *Continued*

Analyte or Test	Criteria for Acceptable Performance
Chemistry Laboratory *(cont.)*	
Bilirubin (total)	Target value +/− 0.4 mg/dL or +/− 20% (greater)
Blood gas pO_2	Target value +/− 3 SD
pCO_2	Target value +/− 5 mm Hg or +/− 8% (greater)
pH	Target value +/− 0.04
Calcium, total	Target value +/− 1.0 mg/dL
Chloride	Target value +/− 5%
Cholesterol, total	Target value +/− 10%
Cholesterol, HDL	Target value +/− 30%
Creatine kinase	Target value +/− 30%
Creatine kinase isoenzymes	MB elevated (presence or absence) or target value +/− 3 SD
Creatine	Target value +/− 0.3 mg/dL or +/− 15% (greater)
Glucose (excluding waived glucose methods)	Target value +/− 6 mg/dL or 10% (greater)
Iron, total	Target value +/− 20%
LDH	Target value +/− 20%
LDH isoenzymes	LDH1/LDH2 (+ or −) or target value +/− 30%
Magnesium	Target value +/− 25%
Potassium	Target value +/− 0.5 mmol/L
Sodium	Target value +/− 4 mmol/L
Total protein	Target value +/− 10%
Triglycerides	Target value +/− 25%
Urea nitrogen	Target value +/− 2 mg/dL or +/− 9% (greater)
Uric acid	Target value +/− 17%
Endocrinology	
Cortisol	Target value +/− 25%
Free thyroxine	Target value +/− 3 SD
HCG	Target value +/− 3 SD, positive or negative
T3 Uptake	Target value +/− 3 SD
Triiodothyronine	Target value +/− 3 SD
Thyroid stimulating hormone	Target value +/− 3 SD
Thyroxine	Target value +/− 20% or 1.0 mg/dL (greater)

Continued

APPENDIX D *Continued*

Analyte or Test	Criteria for Acceptable Performance
Toxicology	
Alcohol, blood	Target value +/− 25%
Blood lead	Target value +/− 10% or 4 mcg/dL (greater)
Carbamazepine	Target value +/− 25%
Digoxin	Target value +/− 20% or +/− 2 ng/mL (greater)
Ethosuximide	Target value +/− 20%
Gentamicin	Target value +/− 25%
Lithium	Target value +/− 0.3 mmol/L or +/− 20% (greater)
Phenobarbital	Target value +/− 20%
Phenytoin	Target value +/− 25%
Primidone	Target value +/− 25%
Procainamide (and metabolite)	Target value +/− 25%
Quinidine	Target value +/− 25%
Tobramycin	Target value +/− 25%
Theophylline	Target value +/− 25%
Valproic acid	Target value +/− 25%
Hematology	
Cell identification	90% or greater consensus on ID
WBC differential	Target value +/− 3 SD based on the percentage of different types of WBCs in the sample
Erythrocyte count	Target value +/− 6%
Hematocrit (excluding spun Hcts)	Target value +/− 6%
Hemoglobin	Target value +/− 7%
Leukocyte count	Target value +/− 15%
Platelet count	Target value +/− 25%
Fibrinogen	Target value +/− 20%
Partial thromboplastin time	Target value +/− 15%
Prothrombin time	Target value +/− 15%
Immunohematology	
ABO grouping	100% accuracy
D (Rho) typing	100% accuracy
Unexpected antibody detection	80% accuracy
Compatibility testing	100% accuracy
Antibody identification	80% accuracy

From 57 CFR: Clinical Laboratory Improvement Amendment of 1988: Final Rule. U.S. Government Printing Office, Washington, DC, 1988.

Answers to Practice Problems

PRACTICE TEST 1

1. 50
2. −56
3. 107
4. 4
5. 19
6. 40
7. −18
8. 9
9. 8
10. 71
11. 8.7
12. 1¼
13. 4⁷/₂₄
14. ⁹/₁₀
15. ¹/₁₆
16. 3¹/₃
17. 5⁵/₈
18. 75%
19. 0.75
20. 520 mg
21. 0.0025 g
22. 0.250 L
23. 5
24. 0.453 kg
25. 165 cm
26. ¹/₅ dilution
27. 10
28. SV = 100 µL, DV = 400 µL
29. 333 mL
30. 500 mL

PRACTICE TEST 2

1. 19
2. −8
3. 68
4. 11
5. 23
6. 30
7. −32
8. 10.8
9. 4
10. 312
11. 9
12. 1
13. 4¹/₂₄
14. 1¹/₆
15. ¹/₈
16. 3¹/₂
17. 3³/₄
18. 0.83
19. 0.75
20. 390 mg
21. 0.125 g
22. 0.150 L
23. 10 mL

24. 75 kg
25. 183 cm
26. ⅕ dilution
27. 5
28. SV = 100 μL, DV = 900 μL
29. 250 mL
30. 200 mL

PRACTICE TEST 3

1. Take medication as needed
2. Take medication every day
3. Take medication before meals
4. Subcutaneous
5. Take medication every morning
6. ½ scored tablet
7. 2 tablets
8. 3 tablets
9. 0.75 g/day
10. 60 mL/day
    20 mL/dose

PRACTICE TEST 4

1. Take medication three times a day
2. Take medication two times a day
3. Immediately
4. Nothing by mouth
5. Drops
6. 2 tablets
7. 2 tablets
8. 2 tablets
9. 850 mg/day
10. 5 mL

PRACTICE TEST 5

1. 7.5 mmol/L with K^+
   3 mmol/L without K^+
2. 318 mOsm/kg

3. 43 mOsm/kg
4. 119.7 mL/min
5. MCV = 91 fL
   MCH = 37 pg
   MCHC = 42%
6. 35,000 CFU/mL
   Possible but not probable
7. Mean   = 4
   Median = 4
   Mode   = 4
8. 95%
9. ±1 SD = 95–105 mg/dL
   ±2 SD = 90–110 mg/dL
   ±3 SD = 85–115 mg/dL
10. Analyzer A

PRACTICE TEST 6

1. 16 mmol/L with K^+
   11 mmol/L without K^+
2. 265 mOsm/kg
3. 91 mOsm/kg
4. 66.1 mL/min
5. MCV = 94 fL
   MCH = 31 pg
   MCHC = 33%
6. 7000 CFU/mL
   No
7. Mean   = 26
   Median = 25.5
   Mode   = 25
8. Probability = 66.7%
9. ±1 SD = 235–265 mg/dL
   ±2 SD = 220–280 mg/dL
   ±3 SD = 205–295 mg/dL
10. Analyzer B

CHAPTER 1

1. 32
2. 19

3. 37

4. 14

5. −18

6. −54

7. −91

8. −70

9. −11

10. −27

11. 0

12. 60

13. 7

14. −10

15. −56

16. 4

17. 156

18. 84

19. 66

20. 7

21. 10

22. +5, not −5. Remember, two negatives make a positive.

23. 11

24. −21

25. −2

26. 0.629

27. 12.7

28. 4.99

29. 6.67

30. 5.56

31. 3.64

32. 2.82

CHAPTER 2

1. 926.9 contains four significant figures.

2. 707 contains three significant figures.

3. 123.06 contains five significant figures.

Remember that the 0 is significant since it is contained within the number.

4. 0.0402 contains three significant figures. Only the digits 402 are significant; the digits 0.0 are not significant.

5. 0.82610 contains five significant figures. The 0 that follows the 1 is significant, while the 0 that precedes the 8 is not.

6. 338.00 contains five significant figures. Zeroes to the right of a decimal point are considered to be significant.

7. The answer to the problem is 358.9, not 358.93 because the final answer can only have one digit to the right of the decimal point, as three of the four numbers in the calculation are precise only to the first decimal place.

8. The answer is 97.5.

9. $125.957 - 31.22 = 94.74$. The final answer can be precise only to the one-one-hundredth position.

10. The answer is 0.027.

11. The answer is 524, not 524.52, since the final answer can have only three significant figures.

12. 4.043 is the answer.

13. 3.9 is the answer, not 3.91, since the final answer can have only two significant figures.

14. The answer is 4.1.

15. 0.682

16. 12.8

17. 4.16

18. 3.34

19. 5.56

20. 2.64

21. 7.82

22. 9.365×10^3

23. 7.120×10^2

24. 2.0000×10^3

25. 2.541×10^{-1}

26. 8.22×10^{-4}

27. 4.77×10^{-6}

28. 4.05×10^6. Using the rule (rule 3) for multiplication with exponents, $[(b \times 10^a)(c \times 10^d)] = (bc)^{a+d}$, and substituting into it the numbers from the problem, the following equation is derived: $[(9.62)(4.21)]^{3+2} = 4.05 \times 10^6$.

29. 1.75×10^6

30. 6.62×10^{-1}. Using the rule (rule 3) for multiplication with exponents, the following equation was derived: $[(6.91)(9.58)]^{-3+1}$, which equals 66.2×10^{-2}. 66.2×10^{-2} can be expressed as 6.62×10^{-1}. This can be verified by solving the problem without using scientific notation. $6.91 \times 10^{-3} = 0.00691$ and $9.58 \times 10^1 = 95.8$. Multiplying 0.00691×95.8 yields 0.662 or 6.62×10^{-1}.

31. 5.46×10^{-5}

32. 3.0×10^7. Using the rule (rule 4) for multiplying a number in scientific notation by an exponent, the following equation is derived: $[(5.5)(5.5)]^{(3)(2)}$, which equals 30.2×10^6. This equation can also be expressed as 3.0×10^7.

33. 3.6×10^{19}

34. 5.9×10^{-3}

35. 4.9×10^{-9}

36. 2.8×10^2. Using the division rule (rule 5), the following equation is derived:

$$\frac{8.6 \times 10^4}{3.1 \times 10^2} = \frac{8.6 \times 10^{4-2}}{3.1} = 2.8 \times 10^2$$

37. 2.6

38. 5.091

39. 4.2×10^{-2}

40. 2.92×10^2

41. 3.6×10^{-2}

42. 3.9×10^3

43. 2.9×10^{-2}

1. The numerator is the top number of a fraction, and the denominator is the bottom number of the fraction. Therefore, in the fraction $1/2$, 1 is the numerator and 2 is the denominator.

2. The numerator is 5 and the denominator is 6.

3. The numerator is 4 and the denominator is 6.

4. The numerator is 1 and the denominator is 3.

5. Reducing fractions to their simplest form means changing the numerator and the denominator so that they cannot be divided by whole numbers, or in other words, making them as simple as they can be. To reduce a fraction to its simplest form, a number that is common to both the numerator and the denominator must be determined. In this fraction, $5/25$, the denominator is divisible by the numerator; therefore, 5 is the common number. If both parts of the fraction are divided by 5, the fraction is simplified to $1/5$. Note that when a fraction is simplified, the overall value, or ratio, of the fraction does not change.

6. The fraction $4/8$ can be reduced to its simplest form of $1/2$.

7. The fraction $2/6$ can be reduced to $1/3$.

8. The fraction $6/30$ can be reduced to $1/5$.

9. The common denominator is the number common to both parts of the fraction. In this case, the common denominator must be determined for the fractions $3/4$ and $2/3$. The simplest method is to multiply the denominators to form a common denominator. Then the numerators of both fractions must be changed as well by multiplying each numerator by the number used to convert the denominator of each fraction into the common denominator. For example, the common denominator of $3/4$ and $2/3$ is 12. Therefore, the denominators of both fractions become 12. Since 4 was multiplied by 3 to become the common denominator 12, the numerator of the fraction must also be multiplied by 3. This changes the fraction from $3/4$ to $9/12$. The same process is used on the fraction $2/3$, which becomes $8/12$.

10. The common denominator of these fractions is 6. The fraction $5/6$ remains unchanged, but the fraction $1/2$ becomes $3/6$.

11. Before addition can be performed, a common denominator for $1/2$ and $3/4$ must be determined. The common denominator for these fractions is 4, and the fraction $1/2$ is converted into the fraction $2/4$. Now the addition calculation can be performed by adding the numerators of the fractions. Therefore, $2/4$ plus $3/4$ equals $5/4$. The fraction $5/4$ must be reduced to its lowest form, $1 1/4$.

12. $6/8$ or $3/4$

13. $1 3/10$

14. $11/15$

15. $2/5$

16. $5/12$

17. $5/8$

18. $1/4$

19. When fractions are multiplied, the numerators are multiplied together and the denominators are multiplied together. Therefore, the product of this equation is $2/15$.

20. $28/40$ or $7/10$

21. $1/4$

22. $2/6$ or $1/3$

23. To divide fractions, the fraction to the right of the division sign is inverted and the two fractions are multiplied together. In this problem, the fraction $1/4$ is inverted to $4/1$ and multiplied by $1/3$ to yield $4/3$. This fraction is reduced to its lowest term, $1 1/3$.

24. $18/15$ or $1 1/5$

25. When performing calculations using mixed fractions, i.e., fractions with a combination of whole numbers and fractions, the same rules (e.g., for multiplication or division) apply to the fraction portion of the number. Therefore, in this example, a common denominator for the fractions $2/3$ and $3/8$ must be determined. In this case, the common denominator is 24. Therefore, the fractions are converted into $16/24$ and $9/24$. Since this is an addition calculation, the numerators of the fractions are added together for a sum of $25/24$. Next, the whole numbers are added together for a sum of 3. Together the fraction becomes $3 25/24$. Since this fraction is not in its simplest form, it must be reduced to the final answer of $4 1/24$.

26. $6 1/12$

27. $1 1/15$

28. $13/24$

29. To multiply or divide mixed fractions, each fraction must first be converted into its compound form by multiplying the whole number of the fraction by the denominator and adding the numerator to that sum. Once the fractions have been converted into their compound form, the multiplication or division calculations can be performed. In this problem, $2 4/5$ is

converted into its compound form of $^{14}/_5$, and $1^5/_6$ is converted into its compound form of $^{11}/_6$. Next, these fractions are multiplied to yield a product of $^{154}/_{30}$, which is simplified to its final form of $5^2/_{15}$.

30. $3^1/_3$

31. $1^7/_{12}$

32. $1^{13}/_{15}$

33. To convert a fraction into a decimal, divide the numerator by the denominator. In this case, 2 is divided by 3 for an answer of 0.67.

34. 0.83

35. 0.50

36. To convert a decimal to a percentage, multiply the decimal by 100. A shortcut method is to move the decimal point two spaces to the right. In this problem, 0.75 becomes 75%.

37. 22%

38. 10%

39. This problem is solved by using ratio and proportion and the following formula:

$$\frac{\text{What you want}}{\text{What you have}} \times \text{Drug form (DF)}$$

$$= \text{Amt. of dispensed drug (ADD)}$$

In this case, you want a 0.50 mg dose of a drug, and you have the drug in 0.25 mg tablet form. Because the drug is dispensed in a tablet, the DF value is a tablet. Therefore:

$$\frac{0.50}{0.25} \times 1 \text{ tablet} = 2$$

The nurse practitioner would give the patient two 0.25 mg tablets for the correct dose.

40. The pharmacist gave the patient one-half of the scored 500 mg tablet to equal a dose of 250 mg.

CHAPTER 4

1. 25.5×10^{-6} g or 2.55×10^{-5} g

2. 3.0×10^{-2} L

3. 750 cm

4. 1.0×10^4 m

5. 100 dL

6. 15×10^{-6} mm

7. 226.4 g. To determine the number of grams, multiply the number of ounces by the conversion factor 28.3.

8. 1.83 m

9. 948 mL

10. 3.79 L

11. 250 mg/L

12. 0.4 mg/L

13. 1200 mg/dL

14. 2.5 g/L

15. The answer is 2×10^4 mm^2 or 20,000 mm^2. Since 1 mm is 100 times smaller than 1 cm, 1 mm^2 is 100×100 or 10,000 times smaller than 1 cm^2. Since there was 2 cm^2, 10,000 is multiplied by 2.

16. 95°F

17. 24.8°F

18. 98.8°C

19. −20.6°C

CHAPTER 5

1. An SV of 4 mL added to 12 mL of diluent is a $^1/_4$ dilution. This is because the SV of 4 mL is diluted into a TV of 16 mL. Therefore, the dilution factor is 4.

2. An SV of 0.5 mL added to 2 mL of diluent is a $^1/_5$ dilution. This is because the SV of 0.5 mL is diluted into a TV of 2.5 mL. Therefore, the dilution factor is 5.

3. $^1/_{20}$ dilution, dilution factor of 20.

4. $^1/_5$ dilution, dilution factor of 5.

5. The final dilution is $\frac{1}{16}$. $\frac{1}{2} \times \frac{1}{2} \times \frac{1}{4} = \frac{1}{16}$.

6. The final dilution factor is 16.

7. The dilution factor for tube 2 is 4 ($\frac{1}{2} \times \frac{1}{2} = \frac{1}{4}$). Since the original concentration was 100, 100 ÷ 4, or 25, is the concentration of tube 2.

8. The dilution factor for tube 1 is 2.

9. The dilution in which the last positive reaction occurred was the $\frac{1}{8}$ dilution. Therefore, the patient's CMV antibody titer is 8.

10. In the first well, the serum is diluted $\frac{1}{5}$, in the second well $\frac{1}{25}$, in the third well $\frac{1}{100}$, in the fourth well $\frac{1}{400}$, in the fifth well $\frac{1}{1600}$, and in the sixth well $\frac{1}{6400}$.

CHAPTER 6

1. A 15% w/w solution is prepared by adding 15 g of solute to 85 g of solvent. Usually in the health care field, the solvent is either water (in deionized, distilled, or sterile form), saline, or a buffer. Percent w/w solutions are defined as 1 g of solute per 100 g of solvent.

2. A 15% w/v solution is prepared by adding 15 g of solute in 85 mL of solvent.

3. A 15% v/v solution is prepared by adding 15 mL of solute in 85 mL of solvent.

4. In this problem, 10 mL of bleach are needed to prepare a 10% v/v solution, and 90 mL of deionized water would be used as the solvent.

5. There would be 10 g of NaOH dissolved in a 10% w/v solution.

6. This problem is solved using ratio and proportion. By definition, a 20% w/v KCl solution contains 20 g of KCl dissolved in 100 mL of solvent. The problem asks for the number of grams of KCl per 10 mL of this solution. Therefore:

$$\frac{20 \text{ g KCl}}{100 \text{ mL solvent}} = \frac{X \text{ g KCl}}{10 \text{ mL solvent}}$$
$$(20)(10) = 100X$$
$$200 = 100X$$
$$2 = X$$

Therefore, there are 2 g of KCl for every 10 mL of this solution.

7. This problem can be solved by using the following formula:
$$C_1V_1 = C_2V_2$$
where $C_1 = 75\%$, $V_1 = X$, $C_2 = 25\%$, and $V_2 = 500$ mL. Therefore:
$$(75)(X) = (25)(500)$$
$$75X = 12{,}500$$
$$X = \frac{12{,}500}{75}$$
$$= 166.7$$

Therefore, 167 mL of 75% EtOH are placed in a 500 mL container and qs'd to the 500 mL mark (or 333 mL of diluent are added to 167 mL of 75% EtOH to make 500 mL of 25% EtOH).

8. In this equation, $C_1 = 20\%$, $V_1 = 300$ mL, $C_2 = X$, and $V_2 = 1000$ mL.
$$(20)(300) = (X)(1000)$$
$$6000 = 1000X$$
$$\frac{6000}{1000} = X$$
$$6 = X$$

Therefore, the new Tris buffer solution has a concentration of 6%.

CHAPTER 7

1. Medication is taken three times a day.

2. Sublingual

3. Medication is taken two times a day.

4. Medication is taken as needed.

5. By mouth

6. Every 4 hours

7. Using the following formula:
$$\frac{\text{What you want}}{\text{What you have}} \times \text{Drug form} = \text{ADD}$$
the following equation is derived:
$$\frac{250 \text{ mg}}{125 \text{ mg}} \times 1 \text{ caplet} = \text{ADD}$$
$$2 \text{ caplets} = \text{ADD}$$
Two caplets would be dispensed.

8. One-half of the 1000 mg tablet.

9. Four of the 25 mg tablets would be dispensed.

10. 0.5 mL cough medicine would be dispensed.

CHAPTER 8

1. The patient would be given two tablets every 4 hours.

2. The patient would be given two tablets each day.

3. The patient would be given 3300 mg/day or 3.3 g/day of drug Y.

4. The patient would be given 22 g/day of drug B.

5. There are 5 mL in a teaspoon.

6. There are 15 mL in a tablespoon.

7. 20 mL administered in 5 mL dosages (1 teaspoon) four times a day.

8. 750 mg of drug C is administered.

9. 6600 mg, or 6.6 g of the drug, is administered per day.

10. 50 gtt/min

11. 6 mL/hr

12. 1.45 mg of the drug is administered.

CHAPTER 9

1. The anion gap is calculated by subtracting the concentrations of chloride and bicarbonate from the sodium concentration. Some laboratories include the potassium concentration among the cations that are measured. The anion gap for this problem without potassium in the calculation is 13 mmol/L, and without potassium the anion gap is 17 mmol/L.

2. 3 without potassium, 6 with potassium.

3. 1 without potassium, 3 with potassium.

4. 21 without potassium, 28 with potassium.

5. The serum osmolality is calculated by the following formula:
Calculated osmolality (mOsmol/kg H_2O)
$$= 1.86 [Na^+] + \frac{[\text{glucose}]}{18} + \frac{[\text{BUN}]}{2.8}$$
$$= (1.86)(147) + \frac{110}{18} + \frac{15}{2.8}$$
$$= 273.4 + 6.1 + 5.4$$
$$= 285 \text{ mOsmol/kg } H_2O$$

6. 271 mOsmol/kg H_2O

7. 305 mOsmol/kg H_2O

8. 315 mOsmol/kg H_2O

9. The osmolal gap is the difference between measured osmolality and calculated osmolality. The calculated osmolality for this problem is 287 mOsm/kg, and the measured osmolality is 290 mOsm/kg. Therefore, the osmolal gap = $290 - 287 = 3$ mOsm/kg H_2O.

10. 16 mOsm/kg H_2O

11. 12 mOsm/kg H_2O

12. 2 mOsm/kg H_2O

13. The concentration of LDL cholesterol can be calculated with the following formula:
$$\text{LDL chol.} = \text{Total chol.} - \left(\text{HDL chol.} + \frac{\text{Trig}}{5} \right)$$
$$= 195 \text{ mg/dL} - \left(45 \text{ mg/dL} + \frac{150}{5} \right)$$
$$= 195 - 75$$
$$= 120 \text{ mg/dL}$$

14. 179 mg/dL

15. 83 mg/dL

16. 212 mg/dL

CHAPTER 10

1. Using ratio and proportion, the following equation is derived:
$$\frac{25 \text{ mEq}}{1000 \text{ mL}} = \frac{X \text{ mEq}}{950 \text{ mL}}$$
Cross-multiplying the equation yields:
$$(25)(950) = (1000)(X)$$
$$23{,}750 = 1000X$$
$$24 = X$$
The sodium concentration can be expressed as 24 mEq/950 mL.

2. To solve this problem, first convert deciliters into milliliters.
$$\frac{65 \text{ mg}}{100 \text{ mL}} = \frac{X \text{ mg}}{1350 \text{ mL}}$$
Cross-multiplying the equation yields:
$$(65)(1350) = (100)(X)$$
$$87{,}750 = 100X$$
$$X = 878 \text{ mg}/1350 \text{ mL}$$

3. $$\frac{525 \text{ mg}}{100 \text{ mL}} = \frac{X \text{ mg}}{1345 \text{ mL}}$$
$$(525)(1345) = (100)(X)$$
$$706{,}125 = 100X$$
$$X = 7061 \text{ mg or } 7.1 \text{ g}/1345 \text{ mL}$$

4. The value of 1000 mg/2240 mL is comparable to 1000 mg/24 hours since the collection period and volume are interchangeable.

5. 40 mEq/12 hr.

6. The amount of urine in mL/min is equal to 2432 mL/1440 min or 1.69 mL/min. Using the clearance formula:
$$\text{Clearance} = \frac{(188 \text{ mg/dL})(1.69 \text{ mL/min})}{1.8 \text{ mg/dL}}$$
$$= 176 \text{ mL/min}$$

7. The corrected clearance value is calculated by accounting for the patient's body size. From Figure 10-1, the patient's body size is 1.58 m². Since

the clearance test is based on a body surface area of 1.73 m², the calculated clearance is multiplied by the product of 1.73 divided by 1.58:
Corrected clearance
$$= 176 \text{ mL/min} \times \frac{1.73 \text{ m}^2}{1.58 \text{ m}^2}$$
$$= 176 \text{ mL/min} \times 1.09$$
$$= 192 \text{ mL/min}$$

8. The rate of urine production is calculated to be 1.17 mL/min. Using the clearance formula:
$$\text{Clearance} = \frac{(117 \text{ mg/dL})(1.17 \text{ mL/min})}{2.3 \text{ mg/dL}}$$
$$= 60 \text{ mL/min}$$

9. The corrected clearance is calculated by adjusting the patient's body surface area. From the nomogram in Figure 10-1, the patient's surface area is 1.80 m². Therefore, the corrected clearance is:
Corrected clearance
$$= 60 \text{ mL/min} \times \frac{1.73 \text{ m}^2}{1.80 \text{ m}^2}$$
$$= 60 \times 0.96$$
$$= 58 \text{ mL/min}$$

10. The temperature difference between the calibrated temperature, 16°C, and the urine temperature, 4°C, is 12°C. For every 3°C below 16°C, 0.001 must be subtracted from the result. Since the difference is 12°C, 12 is divided by 3 to derive the amount by which 0.001 should be multiplied: $^{12}/_{3}$ = 4. Therefore, 0.004 should be subtracted from the obtained value of 1.027, resulting in a corrected specific gravity of 1.023.

11. The specific gravity of 1.025 must have 0.002 subtracted from the reading to correct for the colder temperature. Thus, the correct specific gravity is 1.023.

12. For every 3°C above 16°C, 0.001 must be added to the specific gravity result. The difference between 16°C and 32°C is 16,

and $^{16}/_3$ is approximately 5.0. Therefore, 0.001 is added five times to the obtained specific gravity result. Thus the corrected specific gravity is 1.018.

13. The specific gravity is adjusted upward by 0.003, resulting in a corrected specific gravity of 1.007.

14. For every g/dL of protein, the specific gravity is falsely elevated by 0.001. Since there is 2 g/dL of protein in this sample, the effect is a false elevation of 0.002. Therefore, the correct specific gravity is 1.023.

15. The corrected specific gravity is 1.028.

16. For every g/dL of glucose, the specific gravity is falsely elevated by 0.004. Since the urine contains 3 g/dL of glucose, the specific gravity is falsely elevated by 0.012. Therefore, the correct specific gravity is 1.026.

17. The corrected specific gravity is 1.010.

CHAPTER 11

1. The MCV (fL) is calculated from the following formula:
$$MCV\ (fL) = \frac{Hct \times 10}{RBC\ count}$$
Substituting into the formula the data from the problem yields:
$$MCV\ (fL) = \frac{21 \times 10}{3.2}$$
$$= 66\ fL$$

2. MCV = 100

3. MCV = 122

4. The formula for MCH is:
$$MCH\ (pg) = \frac{Hemoglobin\ (g/dL) \times 10}{RBC\ count\ (million\ per\ \mu L)}$$
Substituting into the formula the data from the problem yields:
$$MCH\ (pg) = \frac{10\ g/dL \times 10}{3.0\ (million\ per\ \mu L)}$$
$$= 33\ pg$$

5. MCH = 49 pg

6. MCH = 42 pg

7. The mean MCHC is calculated by the following formula:
$$MCHC\ (\%) = \frac{Hb\ (g/dL) \times 100}{Hematocrit\ (\%)}$$
Substituting into the formula the data from the problem yields:
$$MCHC\ (\%) = \frac{16\ (g/dL) \times 100}{36\ (\%)}$$
$$= 44\%$$

8. MCHC = 33%

9. MCHC = 33%

10. The factor method for counting WBCs uses the following information:
Factor = 1/area × depth factor × dilution factor
Area counted = number of large squares counted
Depth factor = reciprocal of depth $[1/(^1/_{10})] = 10$
Dilution factor = reciprocal of dilution $[1/(^1/_{20})] = 20$
Therefore, the factor is:
$$\frac{1}{4} \times 10 \times 20 = 50$$
Multiply the number of WBCs counted by the factor to determine the WBC count/mm^3: $74 \times 50 = 3,700/mm^3$

11. WBC count = 7250/mm^3

12. WBC count = 4600/mm^3

13. The factor method for RBC counts is similar to that used for WBC counts. The same formula is used, except that the dilution and area are different. Therefore, the factor for RBC counts is:
$$Factor = \frac{1}{0.2} \times 10 \times 200 = 10,000$$
Multiplying the number of RBCs counted by the factor yields the RBC count/mm^3: $487 \times 10,000 = 4.87 \times 10^6/mm^3$

14. RBC count = $2.69 \times 10^6/mm^3$

15. RBC count = $6.15 \times 10^6/mm^3$

16. Platelet count = 222,000/mm^3

17. Platelet count = 68,000/mm^3

18. Platelet count = 142,000/mm^3

19. WBC count = 1950/mm³. This is calculated using the formula:

$$\#Cells/mm^3 = \frac{\# \text{ Cells counted} \times \text{depth factor} \times \text{dilution factor}}{\text{Area counted}}$$

In this problem, 78 cells were counted, the depth factor is 10, the dilution factor is 10, and the area counted is 4.

20. 3000 WBC/mm³

21. 1.6 × 10⁶ RBC/mm³

22. 1.2 × 10⁶ RBC/mm³

23. 98,500 platelets/mm³

24. 16,500 platelets/mm³

25. The formula used to calculate reticulocytes is:

$$\frac{\# \text{ Reticulocytes counted per 1000 erythrocytes}}{1000} \times 100$$

Using the formula and substituting into the data from the problem:

$$\frac{46}{1000} \times 100 = 4.6\% \text{ reticulocyte count}$$

26. 1.8% reticulocyte count

27. The formula used to calculate the number of reticulocytes using the Miller disc is:

$$\frac{\# \text{ Reticulocytes in small and large squares}}{(\# \text{ RBCs in square 2})(9)} \times 100$$

Substituting into the equation the data from the problem:

$$\frac{65 \text{ reticulocytes}}{(208 \text{ RBCs})(9)} \times 100 = 3.5\% \text{ reticulocyte count}$$

28. 2.2% reticulocyte count

29. Six vials of RhIG should be given. The calculation results in a value of 4.8. The result is rounded to the nearest whole number, 5, and an extra vial is given as an extra precaution.

30. Three vials of RhIG are given.

CHAPTER 12

1. 135,500 CFU/mL

2. 16,900 CFU/mL

3. 134,000 CFU/mL

4. 7000 CFU/mL

5. When the concentration is between 1000 and 100,000 organisms, there is a possible urinary tract infection.

6. A CFU count above 100,000/mL indicates a probable urinary tract infection. A CFU count below 1000/mL indicates contamination of a clean-catch urine sample.

7. Tube 10

CHAPTER 13

1. 48

2. 48.5

3. The modal number is 49.

4. The variance for this set of numbers is 2.66.

5. The standard deviation is the square root of the variance, 2.7, or 1.6.

6. The CV is 3.4%.

7. The mean is 428 mg/dL.

8. The median glucose value is 429 mg/dL.

9. The modal value is 430 mg/dL. Note that this set of numbers does not have a Gaussian distribution, as the mean, median, and modal numbers are not the same.

10. The variance is 4.23 mg²/dL².

11. The standard deviation is 2.1 mg/dL, or the square root of 4.23 mg²/dL². Note that the units for the standard deviation are the same as the units for the data values.

12. The CV for this set of glucose values is 0.5%.

13. There is approximately a 67% probability that a control result will fall within ±1 standard deviation of the mean.

14. 95.5% probability

15. 99.7% probability

16. 4.5% probability

17. 0.03% probability

18. The ± 2 standard deviation range includes all values between 9.5 and 15.5.

19. The ± 3 standard deviation range for this group of data is from 193.5 to 256.5.

CHAPTER 14

1. A shift occurs when six or seven consecutive control values fall on the same side of the mean.

2. A trend occurs when six or seven consecutive control values steadily increase or decrease in value.

3. Some examples of preanalytical errors are incorrect anticoagulant used, improper mixing of anticoagulant, and specimen identification problems.

4. Some examples of analytical errors are instrument not calibrated, pipetting errors, and instrument malfunction.

5. Some examples of postanalytical errors are charting results on the wrong patient chart and making transcribing errors.

6. The 1_{2s} rule is a warning rule.

7. The 1_{3s} rule is usually violated because of random error.

8. The 2_{2s} rule is usually violated because of systematic error.

9. The R_{4s} rule is violated when there is a spread or range of more than 4 standard deviations between the results

for each level of quality control. For example, if the result for one level of control is $+2.2$ standard deviations from the mean while the other control result is -2.1 standard deviations from the mean, the range or spread between them is 4.3 standard deviations, exceeding 4 standard deviations. This rule is generally violated because of random error.

10. The 4_{1s} rule is violated if one level of control exceeds ± 1 standard deviation for four consecutive runs or if both levels of control exceeds ± 2 standard deviations for two consecutive runs.

11. The 10_x rule is violated if the results for one level of control fall on the same side of the mean for 10 consecutive values or if results for both levels of control fall on the same side of the mean for 5 consecutive values.

CHAPTER 15

1. 98.2%

2. 86.5%

3. 96.0%

4. 97.0%

5. 91.4%

6. $t = -0.538$. Since the tabulated value is 2.093, the null hypothesis is not rejected. Therefore, there is no statistically significant difference between the two analyzers.

7. No, the calculated F value is 1.15, which is below the critical value.

Index

Note: Page numbers in *italics* refer to illustrations; page numbers followed by t refer to tables.